HEART-HEALTHY RECIPE COOKBOOK FOR SENIORS AFTER 50

"Love Your Heart: 30 Days of Delectable Low-Sodium, Low-Fat Goodness for a Vibrant Life!"

Sandra Han Cancel

CONTENTS

INTRODUCTION

Embarking on this journey into the heart's sanctuary feels like stepping onto the dance floor of life, where each beat is a testament to the journey we've trekked through the decades. So, my fellow voyager, get ready for an exploration that's equal parts informative, heartwarming, and, hopefully, a tad heartstring-tugging – the kind that resonates with the symphony of our well-lived years.

In this narrative, your heart takes center stage – a maestro orchestrating the tunes of your life. Picture a heart-healthy diet as the sheet music, guiding the instruments to play in perfect harmony, ensuring your heart dances through life with grace and vigor.

Let's kick off our story with the significance of a heart-healthy diet. It's not just about nutrition; it's about crafting a melody that sustains the vitality of your heart, allowing it to pirouette through the seasons of life with finesse.

As we unravel the basics of heart-healthy eating, think of key nutrients as love letters to your heart – each playing a unique role in composing a symphony of well-being. The dance continues with the waltz of portions – a delicate balancing act that turns your plate into a canvas, a masterpiece of culinary artistry that earns your heart a standing ovation after every meal.

Ever felt like reading food labels is decoding a cryptic crossword puzzle? Fear not, my friend! We're turning it into a thrilling adventure, making you the detective of your own health journey.

Now, let's shift our spotlight to the culinary stage – your kitchen. Imagine it as a theater, and you, the master chef, orchestrating a culinary symphony that nourishes both heart and soul. In this culinary odyssey, we'll explore the art of building a heart-healthy pantry.

The essential ingredients become your stellar cast, taking center stage in your heart-healthy culinary production. Cooking oils and fats are the supporting actors, enhancing the flavor and texture of your culinary masterpiece without stealing the spotlight from your heart's leading role.

Stepping into the grocery store might feel like navigating a bustling marketplace in a foreign land. Worry not! We've got your back with tips and tricks that turn your shopping experience into a delightful adventure, where each item in your cart becomes a treasure trove of heart-healthy goodness.

Now, let's imagine your shopping cart as the conductor's baton, guiding you through aisles where whole grains, lean proteins, colorful vegetables, heart-healthy fruits, and a symphony of nutrient-rich foods await. Each item is a note in the symphony of well-being, creating a harmonious blend that resonates with the beating of your heart.

Dear reader, we get it – this journey may evoke a myriad of emotions. Curiosity, determination, perhaps even a dash of apprehension. We're here with an empathetic ear and a reassuring virtual hand to guide you through. As we continue, let the warmth of our words wrap around you like a comforting embrace, reminding you that you're not alone in this endeavor.

In the upcoming acts, we'll explore the vibrant palette of herbs and spices, dive into the deep blue sea of fish and seafood, savor the richness of low-fat dairy, and embrace the earthiness of legumes and high-fiber foods. We'll even concoct heartwarming soups, seasoned with love, crafted to nourish both body and soul.

And fear not, dear reader, for we shall embark on a 30-day meal plan that transforms the mundane into the extraordinary, making every day a celebration of heart-healthy living. So, fasten your seatbelts and prepare for a gastronomic adventure where health meets humor, and empathy intertwines with expertise.

Let the journey begin!

BASICS OF HEART-HEALTHY EATING

Key Nutrients for Heart Health

Let's begin our exploration with the fundamental building blocks – the key nutrients that serve as the backbone of a heart-healthy diet. Consider these nutrients as the essential players in the symphony of wellness, each contributing to the harmony of a healthy heart.

Omega-3 Fatty Acids: First on our nutritional stage are the omega-3 fatty acids, renowned for their heart-protective qualities. Abundantly found in fatty fish like salmon, mackerel, and trout, as well as in flaxseeds and walnuts, these fats contribute to reducing inflammation, promoting healthy cholesterol levels, and supporting overall cardiovascular health.

Fiber: Enter fiber, the unsung hero in the realm of heart-healthy nutrients. Abundant in whole grains, fruits, vegetables, and legumes, fiber acts as a gentle broom, sweeping through your digestive system, aiding in weight management, and contributing to the regulation of blood sugar and cholesterol levels.

Antioxidants: Picture antioxidants as the guardians of your heart's well-being. Fruits and vegetables of various colors – berries, citrus fruits, spinach, and kale – are rich in these protective compounds. Antioxidants neutralize free radicals, reducing oxidative stress and supporting the longevity of your cardiovascular system.

Potassium: Maintaining a healthy balance of potassium is akin to conducting a steady rhythm for your heart. Found in bananas, sweet potatoes, leafy greens, and citrus fruits, potassium helps regulate blood pressure and fluid balance, crucial elements for heart health.

Calcium: Beyond its role in bone health, calcium also plays a part in maintaining a healthy heart. Low-fat dairy products, fortified plant-based milk, and leafy greens are stellar sources of calcium, supporting muscle function and contributing to cardiovascular well-being.

Portion Control and Balanced Meals

Now, let's explore the art of portion control and the composition of balanced meals – a symphony where each component plays a crucial role, contributing to the melody of a heart-healthy diet.

The Symphony of Portions: Portions are the notes on the culinary sheet music, dictating the harmony of your meal. The practice of portion control is not about deprivation but about moderation. Smaller plates, mindful eating, and savoring each bite are techniques that transform your dining experience into a celebration of well-being.

Balancing Macronutrients: Consider macronutrients – carbohydrates, proteins, and fats – as the trio shaping the nutritional composition of your meals. Opt for complex carbohydrates from whole grains, lean proteins from poultry, fish, and legumes, and healthy fats from sources like avocados and olive oil. This triumvirate ensures a balanced meal that fuels your heart with essential nutrients.

The Plate Method: Visualize your plate as a canvas, and the plate method as the brushstrokes creating a balanced masterpiece. Fill half your plate with colorful vegetables, allocate a quarter to lean proteins, and dedicate the remaining quarter to whole grains. This visual approach ensures a well-rounded and heart-healthy composition.

Reading Food Labels

In the world of heart-healthy eating, the ability to decipher food labels is a skill that empowers you to make informed choices. Let's unravel the mysteries of food labels, turning your grocery shopping into a mindful and health-conscious experience.

Understanding Serving Sizes: The first step in label literacy is comprehending serving sizes. Often, packaged foods present enticing claims, but the serving sizes may differ from what you typically consume. Be vigilant, and use this information to make accurate nutritional assessments.

The Nutrient Breakdown: Venture beyond the calorie count and explore the nutrient breakdown. Keep an eye on saturated and trans fats, cholesterol, sodium, and added sugars. Strive for lower amounts of these components to maintain a heart-healthy balance.

Ingredient List Decoded: Consider the ingredient list as the narrative of your culinary journey. Opt for foods with recognizable, whole ingredients, steering clear of overly processed or heavily refined options. Ingredients listed first are present in higher quantities, guiding you towards healthier choices.

Hidden Sugars and Sodium: Unmasking hidden sugars and sodium is a crucial aspect of label reading. Ingredients with names ending in "ose" often denote sugars, while sodium lurks under various aliases. Revealing these hidden components empowers you to make heart-conscious choices.

As we traverse the landscape of heart-healthy eating, these fundamentals serve as the compass, guiding you toward a nutritional haven. The key nutrients, coupled with the practice of portion control and the ability to decipher food labels, form the bedrock of a heart-healthy lifestyle.

In the subsequent chapters, we'll delve deeper into the nuances of heart-healthy living, exploring the art of building a heart-healthy pantry, crafting whole grains, lean proteins, colorful vegetables, and presenting a 30-day meal plan that transforms your culinary aspirations into a symphony of health and flavor. The journey towards a heart-healthy lifestyle continues, where every meal becomes a note in the melody of well-being.

BUILDING A HEART-HEALTHY PANTRY

Essential Ingredients

Consider essential ingredients as the building blocks of your heart-healthy culinary masterpiece. These are the unsung heroes that lend both flavor and nutritional prowess to your meals, ensuring each bite is a step towards nurturing your heart.

Whole Grains: The cornerstone of a heart-healthy pantry, whole grains bring a plethora of benefits to the table. Think brown rice, quinoa, oats, and whole wheat – these grains pack a punch of fiber, vitamins, and minerals. Their complex carbohydrates release energy gradually, providing sustained fuel for your heart and body.

Lean Proteins: Proteins are the backbone of a well-balanced meal, and opting for lean sources is paramount for heart health. Incorporate skinless poultry, fish, legumes, and plant-based proteins like tofu and tempeh. These choices deliver essential amino acids without the added burden of excessive saturated fats.

Colorful Vegetables: The vibrant hues of vegetables are not just visually appealing; they signify an array of heart-protective nutrients. Dark leafy greens, carrots, bell peppers, and broccoli offer a rich spectrum of vitamins, antioxidants, and fiber. Their presence in your pantry guarantees versatility and nutritional richness in your meals.

Heart-Healthy Fruits: While we often associate fruits with sweetness, they also contribute vital nutrients for heart health. Berries, citrus fruits, apples, and pears bring not only natural sweetness but also a wealth of fiber, vitamins, and antioxidants. Dried fruits, in moderation, can also add a delightful touch to your heart-healthy repertoire.

Healthy Fats: Not all fats are created equal, and your heart benefits from the inclusion of healthy fats. Avocados, nuts, seeds, and olive oil provide monounsaturated and polyunsaturated fats that support heart health. These fats play a role in reducing bad cholesterol levels while promoting the presence of good cholesterol.

Low-Fat Dairy: Dairy can be a valuable source of calcium and protein but opt for low-fat or fat-free varieties to maintain heart health. Greek yogurt, skim milk, and reduced-fat cheese offer the dairy goodness without the saturated fat content that could negatively impact your cardiovascular system.

Cooking Oils and Fats: In the culinary narrative, cooking oils and fats play a significant role in orchestrating flavors while ensuring heart health. Let's delve into the art of choosing the right oils and fats to compose a symphony that aligns with the well-being of your cardiovascular system.

Monounsaturated Fats: Think of monounsaturated fats as the soloists in your culinary symphony. Olive oil, avocado oil, and canola oil are rich in these heart-healthy fats, known for their ability to lower bad cholesterol levels while preserving the integrity of good cholesterol.

Polyunsaturated Fats: The polyunsaturated fats take their turn as supporting instrumentalists, offering a diversity of benefits. Incorporate oils like safflower, sunflower, and flaxseed oil into your pantry, as they contain essential omega-3 and omega-6 fatty acids, contributing to heart health and overall well-being.

Saturated Fats: While a moderate amount of saturated fats is acceptable, it's crucial to exercise caution. Limit sources like butter, lard, and palm oil, as excessive consumption can elevate bad cholesterol levels, potentially impacting cardiovascular health.

Trans Fats: Consider trans fats the discordant notes in your culinary score. Minimize or eliminate sources like partially hydrogenated oils, often found in processed and fried foods. These fats have a detrimental impact on cholesterol levels, making them less than ideal for heart health.

Smart Grocery Shopping Tips

Navigating the aisles of a grocery store can be akin to embarking on a treasure hunt for heart-healthy gems. Let's explore smart grocery shopping tips that ensure your cart is brimming with ingredients conducive to your cardiovascular well-being.

Create a List: Crafting a well-thought-out shopping list is your compass through the grocery store labyrinth. Plan your meals for the week, taking into account essential ingredients and fresh produce, to avoid impulse purchases that may not align with your heart-healthy goals.

Shop the Perimeter: Consider the perimeter of the grocery store your heart-healthy haven. Fresh produce, lean proteins, and dairy are often located along the outer edges, minimizing exposure to processed and less-nutrient-dense options found in the central aisles.

Read Labels Mindfully: Become a detective, scrutinizing labels for hidden ingredients that might sneakily compromise heart health. Pay attention to added sugars, sodium content, and the presence of unhealthy fats. Opt for products with minimal processing and whole, recognizable ingredients.

Explore Whole Foods: Embrace the beauty of whole foods, as nature intended them. Fresh fruits, vegetables, lean meats, and whole grains are not only nutritious but also form the backbone of heart-healthy eating. Minimize reliance on heavily processed or pre-packaged items.

Buy in Bulk: When possible, purchase staple items in bulk. Whole grains, legumes, and nuts can often be more cost-effective when bought in larger quantities. This not only benefits your wallet but also ensures a steady supply of heart-healthy ingredients in your pantry.

UNLOCKING THE BENEFITS OF A LOW-SODIUM LIFE-STYLE

In the realm of nutrition, the impact of sodium on our health is undeniable. Excessive sodium intake has been linked to a range of cardiovascular issues, making it imperative for individuals to embrace a low-sodium lifestyle, particularly for those with heart conditions or those aiming to prevent them. In this exploration, we'll navigate the nuances of low-sodium living, uncovering the benefits, practical strategies, and the flavorful journey toward heart health.

Understanding the Importance of a Low-Sodium Lifestyle:

A low-sodium lifestyle involves consciously limiting the amount of salt in your diet to promote overall health, particularly cardiovascular well-being. Sodium, a vital electrolyte, is necessary for various bodily functions, but excess intake can lead to elevated blood pressure, fluid retention, and increased strain on the heart. For individuals with heart conditions or those looking to prevent them, adopting a low-sodium lifestyle is a proactive step towards better heart health.

Benefits of a Low-Sodium Lifestyle:

1. **Blood Pressure Management:** One of the primary benefits of embracing a low-sodium lifestyle is the positive impact on blood pressure. By reducing sodium intake, individuals can help manage blood pressure levels, lowering the risk of hypertension and its associated complications.

2. **Cardiovascular Health:** A low-sodium diet contributes to overall cardiovascular health. It helps prevent the development of heart conditions, such as coronary artery disease, heart failure, and stroke, providing a protective shield for the heart and blood vessels.

3. **Reduced Fluid Retention:** Sodium has the tendency to cause fluid retention in the body. By adopting a low-sodium lifestyle, individuals can mitigate this effect, promoting better fluid balance and reducing the strain on the cardiovascular system.

4. **Kidney Function Support:** The kidneys play a crucial role in regulating sodium levels in the body. A low-sodium lifestyle can support optimal kidney function, reducing the risk of kidney-related complications and promoting overall renal health.

5. **Improved Weight Management:** High-sodium diets have been associated with increased thirst and a preference for high-calorie, salty foods. By transitioning to a low-sodium lifestyle, individuals can make mindful food choices that support weight management and overall well-being.

Practical Strategies for Embracing a Low-Sodium Lifestyle:

1. **Whole Foods Embrace:** Base your diet on whole, unprocessed foods. Fresh fruits, vegetables, whole grains, and lean proteins

naturally contain lower sodium levels compared to processed alternatives.

2. **Herbs and Spices Mastery:** Elevate the flavor of your dishes with a diverse array of herbs and spices. Experiment with combinations like garlic, basil, thyme, and rosemary to create tantalizing, sodium-free seasonings.

3. **Mindful Label Reading:** Develop the habit of reading food labels diligently. Look out for hidden sources of sodium, such as monosodium glutamate (MSG), sodium nitrate, and sodium benzoate. Opt for products labeled as "low sodium" or "no added salt."

4. **Home Cooking Adventure:** Take charge of your sodium intake by preparing meals at home. This allows you to control the ingredients and seasoning, ensuring that your dishes align with your low-sodium goals.

5. **Gradual Reduction Approach:** If you're accustomed to a higher sodium intake, consider gradually reducing salt in your recipes. This allows your taste buds to adjust, making the transition to a low-sodium lifestyle more manageable and enjoyable.

6. **Smart Dining Out Choices:** When dining out, be proactive in making low-sodium choices. Inquire about preparation methods, request no added salt, and opt for fresh, unprocessed dishes.

Many restaurants are accommodating and can tailor their offerings to suit your dietary preferences.

Navigating the Flavorful Journey:

Contrary to popular belief, a low-sodium lifestyle doesn't equate to bland or tasteless meals. In fact, it opens the door to a world of exciting flavors, textures, and culinary creativity. Here are some tips to make your low-sodium journey delicious:

1. **Citrus Zest:** Harness the bright, zesty flavors of citrus fruits like lemons, limes, and oranges. Grate the zest into your dishes or use the juice as a refreshing marinade.

2. **Vinegar Varieties:** Explore different vinegars, such as balsamic, apple cider, or red wine vinegar, to add depth and acidity to your meals without relying on sodium.

3. **Homemade Stocks:** Prepare sodium-free broths and stocks at home using a variety of herbs, vegetables, and bones. These can serve as flavorful bases for soups, stews, and sauces.

4. **Nut and Seed Crunch:** Introduce texture and a hint of saltiness with a variety of nuts and seeds. Sprinkle them on salads, yogurts, or incorporate them into your favorite dishes.

5. **Dried Herbs:** Stock your pantry with an assortment of dried herbs like thyme, oregano, and basil. These can infuse your recipes with robust flavors without the need for additional salt.

Cautions and Considerations:

While a low-sodium lifestyle offers numerous health benefits, it's essential to approach this journey with awareness and consideration. Some individuals may be more sensitive to sodium reductions, and a drastic change in intake could lead to temporary side effects, such as dizziness or headaches. It's advisable to consult with healthcare professionals or a registered dietitian, especially for those with pre-existing health conditions.

BREAFAST RECIPE

Berry Almond Chia Pudding Parfait

Start your day with a burst of antioxidants and omega-3 fatty acids. This delightful chia pudding parfait is a heart-healthy breakfast that's simple to prepare.

Prep Time: 10 minutes

Cooking Time: No cooking required

Serving Size: 1 parfait

Ingredients:

- 2 tablespoons chia seeds
- 1/2 cup almond milk
- 1/4 teaspoon vanilla extract
- 1/2 cup mixed berries (strawberries, blueberries, raspberries)
- 1 tablespoon sliced almonds
- 1 teaspoon honey (optional)

Instructions:

1. In a bowl, mix chia seeds, almond milk, and vanilla extract. Let it sit for at least 30 minutes or refrigerate overnight until it thickens.
2. Layer the chia pudding with mixed berries in a glass or jar.
3. Top with sliced almonds and drizzle with honey if desired.

Nutritional Information (per parfait):

- Calories: 200
- Protein: 5g

- Carbohydrates: 25g

- Dietary Fiber: 10g

- Fat: 10g

- Saturated Fat: 1g

- Sodium: 20mg

- Potassium: 180mg

- Phosphorus: 120mg

Spinach and Mushroom Egg White Omelet

Packed with protein and vitamins, this egg white omelet is a savory and heart-healthy breakfast option.

Prep Time: 10 minutes

Cooking Time: 5 minutes

Serving Size: 1 omelet

Ingredients:

- 1 cup egg whites

- 1/2 cup fresh spinach, chopped

- 1/4 cup mushrooms, sliced

- 1/4 cup diced tomatoes

- 1 tablespoon feta cheese (optional)

- Salt and pepper to taste

- Cooking spray

Instructions:

1. Heat a non-stick pan over medium heat and coat with cooking spray.

2. Sauté mushrooms until tender, then add spinach and tomatoes. Cook until spinach wilts.

3. Pour egg whites over the vegetables, and sprinkle with feta cheese if desired.

4. Cook until the edges set, then flip and cook the other side.

Nutritional Information (per omelet):

- Calories: 150

- Protein: 25g

- Carbohydrates: 5g

- Dietary Fiber: 1g

- Fat: 3g

- Saturated Fat: 1g

- Sodium: 350mg

- Potassium: 320mg

- Phosphorus: 200mg

Quinoa and Berry Breakfast Bowl

A nutrient-packed bowl with the goodness of quinoa and the sweetness of berries, this breakfast is a delightful combination of flavors and textures.

Prep Time: 15 minutes

Cooking Time: 15 minutes (for quinoa)

Serving Size: 1 bowl

Ingredients:

- 1/2 cup cooked quinoa

- 1/2 cup mixed berries (blueberries, strawberries, blackberries)

- 1 tablespoon slivered almonds

- 1 tablespoon Greek yogurt

- 1 teaspoon honey

Instructions:

1. Cook quinoa according to package instructions.

2. In a bowl, layer quinoa, mixed berries, and slivered almonds.

3. Top with a dollop of Greek yogurt and drizzle with honey.

Nutritional Information (per bowl):

- Calories: 220

- Protein: 8g

- Carbohydrates: 35g

- Dietary Fiber: 6g

- Fat: 6g

- Saturated Fat: 1g

- Sodium: 20mg

- Potassium: 250mg

- Phosphorus: 180mg

Avocado and Tomato Toast

A heart-healthy twist on the classic toast, this recipe adds the creamy goodness of avocado and the freshness of tomatoes.

Prep Time: 10 minutes

Cooking Time: 5 minutes

Serving Size: 1 slice

Ingredients:

- 1 slice whole-grain bread

- 1/2 avocado, mashed
- 1/2 cup cherry tomatoes, sliced
- Salt and pepper to taste
- Fresh cilantro for garnish (optional)

Instructions:

1. Toast the whole-grain bread to your liking.
2. Spread mashed avocado over the toasted bread.
3. Arrange sliced cherry tomatoes on top.
4. Season with salt and pepper, and garnish with fresh cilantro if desired.

Nutritional Information (per slice):

- Calories: 180
- Protein: 4g
- Carbohydrates: 20g
- Dietary Fiber: 8g
- Fat: 10g
- Saturated Fat: 1.5g
- Sodium: 150mg
- Potassium: 470mg
- Phosphorus: 120mg

Blueberry and Almond Overnight Oats

Prepare breakfast the night before with these easy-to-make overnight oats, featuring the sweetness of blueberries and the crunch of almonds.

Prep Time: 5 minutes (plus overnight soaking)

Cooking Time: No cooking required

Serving Size: 1 bowl

Ingredients:

- 1/2 cup rolled oats
- 1/2 cup almond milk
- 1/4 cup fresh blueberries
- 1 tablespoon almond butter
- 1 teaspoon chia seeds
- 1 teaspoon honey (optional)

Instructions:

1. In a jar, combine rolled oats, almond milk, blueberries, almond butter, and chia seeds.
2. Stir well, cover, and refrigerate overnight.
3. In the morning, give it a good mix and drizzle with honey if desired.

Nutritional Information (per bowl):

- Calories: 300
- Protein: 8g
- Carbohydrates: 40g
- Dietary Fiber: 8g
- Fat: 12g
- Saturated Fat: 1g
- Sodium: 80mg
- Potassium: 280mg
- Phosphorus: 220mg

Whole Grain Pancakes with Berries

Enjoy a classic breakfast with a heart-healthy twist. These whole grain pancakes are paired with fresh berries for a delightful morning treat.

Prep Time: 15 minutes

Cooking Time: 10 minutes

Serving Size: 2 pancakes

Ingredients:

- 1/2 cup whole wheat flour
- 1/2 cup almond milk
- 1 egg
- 1 tablespoon Greek yogurt
- 1 teaspoon baking powder
- 1/2 teaspoon vanilla extract
- Mixed berries for topping
- Maple syrup for drizzling (optional)

Instructions:

1. In a bowl, mix whole wheat flour, almond milk, egg, Greek yogurt, baking powder, and vanilla extract.
2. Heat a griddle or non-stick pan over medium heat.
3. Pour batter onto the griddle to make pancakes.
4. Cook until bubbles form, then flip and cook the other side.
5. Top with mixed berries and drizzle with maple syrup if desired.

Nutritional Information (per serving):

- Calories: 280
- Protein: 12g

- Carbohydrates: 40g

- Dietary Fiber: 6g

- Fat: 8g

- Saturated Fat: 1.5g

- Sodium: 180mg

- Potassium: 220mg

- Phosphorus: 150mg

Smoked Salmon and Avocado Bagel

Elevate your breakfast with this elegant and heart-healthy bagel topped with smoked salmon and creamy avocado.

Prep Time: 10 minutes

Cooking Time: No cooking required

Serving Size: 1 bagel

Ingredients:

- 1 whole-grain bagel

- 2 ounces smoked salmon

- 1/2 avocado, sliced

- 1 tablespoon cream cheese (optional)

- Fresh dill for garnish

Instructions:

1. Slice and toast the whole-grain bagel to your liking.

2. Spread cream cheese on the toasted bagel if desired.

3. Layer sliced avocado and smoked salmon on top.

4. Garnish with fresh dill for extra flavor.

Nutritional Information (per bagel):

- Calories: 320
- Protein: 18g
- Carbohydrates: 35g
- Dietary Fiber: 7g
- Fat: 14g
- Saturated Fat: 2.5g
- Sodium: 550mg
- Potassium: 480mg
- Phosphorus: 220mg

Banana Walnut Breakfast Muffins

Enjoy a grab-and-go heart-healthy breakfast with these moist and flavorful banana walnut muffins.

Prep Time: 15 minutes

Cooking Time: 20 minutes

Serving Size: 1 muffin

Ingredients:

- 1 cup whole wheat flour
- 1/2 cup mashed ripe bananas (about 2 medium-sized bananas)
- 1/4 cup chopped walnuts
- 1/4 cup honey
- 1/4 cup unsweetened applesauce
- 1 egg
- 1 teaspoon baking powder
- 1/2 teaspoon cinnamon
- 1/4 teaspoon salt

Instructions:

1. Preheat the oven to 350°F (175°C) and line a muffin tin with paper liners.

2. In a bowl, mix flour, baking powder, cinnamon, and salt.

3. In another bowl, whisk together mashed bananas, honey, applesauce, and egg.

4. Combine the wet and dry ingredients, then fold in chopped walnuts.

5. Spoon the batter into muffin cups and bake for 20 minutes or until a toothpick comes out clean.

Nutritional Information (per muffin):

- Calories: 180
- Protein: 4g
- Carbohydrates: 30g
- Dietary Fiber: 3g
- Fat: 6g
- Saturated Fat: 0.5g
- Sodium: 120mg
- Potassium: 180mg
- Phosphorus: 70mg

Greek Yogurt and Fruit Parfait

Indulge in a delightful Greek yogurt and fruit parfait, combining the richness of yogurt with the sweetness of fresh fruits.

Prep Time: 10 minutes

Cooking Time: No cooking required

Serving Size: 1 parfait

Ingredients:

- 1 cup Greek yogurt
- 1/2 cup mixed berries (strawberries, blueberries, raspberries)
- 1/4 cup granola
- 1 tablespoon honey (optional)

Instructions:

1. In a glass or bowl, layer Greek yogurt, mixed fruits, and granola.
2. Repeat the layers until the container is filled.
3. Drizzle with honey if desired.

Nutritional Information (per parfait):

- Calories: 280
- Protein: 20g
- Carbohydrates: 30g
- Dietary Fiber: 4g
- Fat: 10g
- Saturated Fat: 1g
- Sodium: 80mg
- Potassium: 330mg
- Phosphorus: 250mg

Vegetable and Egg Breakfast Burrito

Fuel your morning with this protein-packed and veggie-filled breakfast burrito, perfect for a satisfying and heart-healthy start to your day.

Prep Time: 15 minutes

Cooking Time: 10 minutes

Serving Size: 1 burrito

Ingredients:

- 1 whole-grain tortilla
- 2 eggs, scrambled
- 1/4 cup black beans, drained and rinsed
- 1/4 cup diced bell peppers
- 1/4 cup diced tomatoes
- 1/4 cup shredded low-fat cheese
- Salsa for topping (optional)
- Fresh cilantro for garnish (optional)

Instructions:

1. In a pan, scramble the eggs until fully cooked.
2. Warm the whole-grain tortilla on a separate pan.
3. Assemble the burrito with scrambled eggs, black beans, bell peppers, tomatoes, and shredded cheese.
4. Fold the sides and roll the burrito.
5. Top with salsa and garnish with fresh cilantro if desired.

Nutritional Information (per burrito):

- Calories: 320
- Protein: 20g

- Carbohydrates: 30g

- Dietary Fiber: 6g

- Fat: 14g

- Saturated Fat: 4g

- Sodium: 450mg

- Potassium: 420mg

- Phosphorus: 250mg

SOUPS

Hearty Lentil and Vegetable Soup

A nourishing soup filled with protein-rich lentils and an array of colorful vegetables. A perfect blend of heartiness and health.

Prep Time: 15 minutes

Cooking Time: 40 minutes

Serving Size: 1.5 cup

Ingredients:

- 1 cup dry green lentils, rinsed
- 1 onion, diced
- 2 carrots, sliced
- 2 celery stalks, chopped
- 3 cloves garlic, minced
- 1 can (14 oz) diced tomatoes, undrained
- 6 cups low-sodium vegetable broth
- 1 teaspoon dried thyme
- 1 teaspoon ground cumin
- Salt and pepper to taste
- 2 cups chopped kale or spinach

Instructions:

1. In a large pot, sauté the diced onion, carrots, celery, and garlic until softened.

2. Add the rinsed lentils, diced tomatoes, vegetable broth, thyme, cumin, salt, and pepper. Bring to a boil.

3. Reduce heat and simmer for 30-35 minutes or until lentils are tender.

4. Stir in the chopped kale or spinach and cook for an additional 5 minutes until wilted.

5. Adjust seasoning if needed and serve hot.

Nutritional Information (per 1.5 cup):

- Calories: 270
- Protein: 18g
- Carbohydrates: 50g
- Dietary Fiber: 18g
- Fat: 1.5g
- Saturated Fat: 0g
- Sodium: 480mg
- Potassium: 980mg
- Phosphorus: 300mg

Tomato Basil Quinoa Soup

A flavorful and protein-packed soup featuring the goodness of quinoa, tomatoes, and fresh basil.

Prep Time: 10 minutes

Cooking Time: 25 minutes

Serving Size: 1 cup

Ingredients:

- 1/2 cup quinoa, rinsed
- 1 onion, finely chopped

- 2 cloves garlic, minced
- 1 can (28 oz) crushed tomatoes
- 4 cups low-sodium vegetable broth
- 1 teaspoon dried oregano
- 1/2 teaspoon dried thyme
- Salt and pepper to taste
- 1/4 cup fresh basil, chopped
- 1 tablespoon olive oil (optional)

Instructions:

1. In a pot, sauté the chopped onion and garlic in olive oil until translucent.

2. Add crushed tomatoes, vegetable broth, rinsed quinoa, oregano, thyme, salt, and pepper. Bring to a boil.

3. Reduce heat and simmer for 15-20 minutes or until quinoa is cooked.

4. Stir in fresh basil just before serving.

5. Adjust seasoning if needed and serve hot.

Nutritional Information (per cup):

- Calories: 180
- Protein: 6g
- Carbohydrates: 30g
- Dietary Fiber: 5g
- Fat: 3g
- Saturated Fat: 0.5g

- Sodium: 420mg

- Potassium: 560mg

- Phosphorus: 150mg

Spinach and White Bean Soup

A light and nutrient-packed soup featuring white beans and spinach, providing a delicious boost of fiber and protein.

Prep Time: 10 minutes

Cooking Time: 20 minutes

Serving Size: 1.5 cup

Ingredients:

- 1 can (15 oz) white beans, drained and rinsed

- 1 onion, diced

- 2 carrots, sliced

- 3 cups fresh spinach, chopped

- 4 cups low-sodium vegetable broth

- 2 cloves garlic, minced

- 1 teaspoon dried rosemary

- 1/2 teaspoon smoked paprika

- Salt and pepper to taste

- 1 tablespoon olive oil (optional)

Instructions:

1. In a pot, sauté the diced onion and garlic in olive oil until softened.

2. Add sliced carrots, white beans, vegetable broth, rosemary, smoked paprika, salt, and pepper. Bring to a simmer.

3. Cook for 15 minutes until carrots are tender.

4. Stir in chopped spinach and cook for an additional 5 minutes until wilted.

5. Adjust seasoning if needed and serve warm.

Nutritional Information (per 1.5 cup):

- Calories: 220
- Protein: 12g
- Carbohydrates: 35g
- Dietary Fiber: 10g
- Fat: 3g
- Saturated Fat: 0.5g
- Sodium: 480mg
- Potassium: 860mg
- Phosphorus: 200mg

Butternut Squash and Red Lentil Soup

A velvety soup combining the sweetness of butternut squash with the protein-rich goodness of red lentils.

Prep Time: 15 minutes

Cooking Time: 30 minutes

Serving Size: 1 cup

Ingredients:

- 2 cups butternut squash, peeled and diced
- 1 cup red lentils, rinsed
- 1 onion, chopped

- 2 cloves garlic, minced
- 1 teaspoon ground cumin
- 1/2 teaspoon ground coriander
- 6 cups low-sodium vegetable broth
- Salt and pepper to taste
- 1 tablespoon olive oil (optional)
- Fresh cilantro for garnish (optional)

Instructions:

1. In a pot, sauté chopped onion and garlic in olive oil until translucent.

2. Add diced butternut squash, red lentils, cumin, coriander, vegetable broth, salt, and pepper. Bring to a boil.

3. Reduce heat and simmer for 25-30 minutes or until butternut squash and lentils are tender.

4. Blend the soup until smooth using an immersion blender or regular blender.

5. Garnish with fresh cilantro before serving.

Nutritional Information (per cup):

- Calories: 230
- Protein: 15g
- Carbohydrates: 45g
- Dietary Fiber: 12g
- Fat: 5g
- Saturated Fat: 1g

- Sodium: 800mg

- Potassium: 950mg

- Phosphorus: 320mg

Minestrone Soup with Whole Wheat Pasta

A classic Italian soup featuring a medley of vegetables and whole wheat pasta, delivering a heart-healthy twist to a beloved dish.

Prep Time: 15 minutes

Cooking Time: 25 minutes

Serving Size: 1.5 cup

Ingredients:

- 1 cup whole wheat pasta, cooked

- 1 can (15 oz) kidney beans, drained and rinsed

- 1 zucchini, diced

- 1 cup green beans, chopped

- 1 onion, finely chopped

- 2 cloves garlic, minced

- 1 can (14 oz) diced tomatoes

- 6 cups low-sodium vegetable broth

- 1 teaspoon dried basil

- 1/2 teaspoon dried oregano

- Salt and pepper to taste

- 1 tablespoon olive oil (optional)

- Grated Parmesan cheese for garnish (optional)

Instructions:

1. In a pot, sauté chopped onion and garlic in olive oil until softened.

2. Add diced zucchini, green beans, diced tomatoes, kidney beans, vegetable broth, basil, oregano, salt, and pepper. Bring to a simmer.

3. Cook for 20 minutes until vegetables are tender.

4. Stir in cooked whole wheat pasta and cook for an additional 5 minutes.

5. Adjust seasoning if needed and garnish with Parmesan cheese before serving.

Nutritional Information (per 1.5 cup):

- Calories: 280
- Protein: 15g
- Carbohydrates: 50g
- Dietary Fiber: 12g
- Fat: 3g
- Saturated Fat: 0.5g
- Sodium: 560mg
- Potassium: 820mg
- Phosphorus: 220mg

Roasted Red Pepper and Chickpea Soup

A robust soup featuring the smokiness of roasted red peppers and the protein-packed goodness of chickpeas.

Prep Time: 15 minutes

Cooking Time: 30 minutes

Serving Size: 1 cup

Ingredients:

- 2 red bell peppers, roasted and diced
- 1 can (15 oz) chickpeas, drained and rinsed
- 1 onion, chopped
- 2 cloves garlic, minced
- 4 cups low-sodium vegetable broth
- 1 teaspoon smoked paprika
- 1/2 teaspoon cayenne pepper
- Salt and pepper to taste
- 1 tablespoon olive oil (optional)
- Fresh parsley for garnish (optional)

Instructions:

1. Roast red bell peppers until charred, then peel, seed, and dice them.

2. In a pot, sauté chopped onion and garlic in olive oil until translucent.

3. Add diced roasted red peppers, chickpeas, vegetable broth, smoked paprika, cayenne pepper, salt, and pepper. Bring to a boil.

4. Reduce heat and simmer for 20-25 minutes.

5. Blend the soup until smooth using an immersion blender or regular blender.

6. Garnish with fresh parsley before serving.

Nutritional Information (per cup):

- Calories: 220

- Protein: 10g

- Carbohydrates: 35g

- Dietary Fiber: 8g

- Fat: 5g

- Saturated Fat: 0.5g

- Sodium: 480mg

- Potassium: 650mg

- Phosphorus: 180mg

Quinoa and Vegetable Stew

A protein-packed stew featuring quinoa and an assortment of colorful vegetables for a wholesome and satisfying meal.

- *Prep Time: 20 minutes*

- *Cooking Time: 35 minutes*

- *Serving Size: 1.5 cups*

Ingredients:

- 1/2 cup quinoa, rinsed

- 1 cup sweet potatoes, diced

- 1 cup carrots, sliced

- 1 cup bell peppers (assorted colors), chopped

- 1 onion, finely chopped

- 2 cloves garlic, minced

- 1 can (15 oz) black beans, drained and rinsed

- 6 cups low-sodium vegetable broth

- 1 teaspoon ground cumin

- 1/2 teaspoon chili powder

- Salt and pepper to taste

- 1 tablespoon olive oil (optional)

- Fresh cilantro for garnish (optional)

Instructions:

1. In a pot, sauté chopped onion and garlic in olive oil until softened.

2. Add diced sweet potatoes, carrots, bell peppers, rinsed quinoa, black beans, vegetable broth, ground cumin, chili powder, salt, and pepper. Bring to a boil.

3. Reduce heat and simmer for 30 minutes or until vegetables are tender.

4. Adjust seasoning if needed and garnish with fresh cilantro before serving.

Nutritional Information (per 1.5 cup):

- Calories: 290

- Protein: 15g

- Carbohydrates: 50g

- Dietary Fiber: 12g

- Fat: 4g

- Saturated Fat: 0.5g

- Sodium: 560mg

- Potassium: 900mg

- Phosphorus: 220mg

Lemon Garlic Orzo Soup

A refreshing and citrusy soup featuring orzo pasta, chickpeas, and a burst of lemon and garlic flavors.

Prep Time: 10 minutes

Cooking Time: 20 minutes

Serving Size: 1 cup

Ingredients:

- 1/2 cup orzo pasta, uncooked

- 1 can (15 oz) chickpeas, drained and rinsed

- 2 cloves garlic, minced

- 1 lemon, juiced and zested

- 4 cups low-sodium vegetable broth

- 1 teaspoon dried thyme

- Salt and pepper to taste

- 1 tablespoon olive oil (optional)

- Fresh parsley for garnish (optional)

Instructions:

1. Cook orzo pasta according to package instructions.

2. In a pot, sauté minced garlic in olive oil until fragrant.

3. Add cooked orzo, chickpeas, vegetable broth, dried thyme, lemon juice, lemon zest, salt, and pepper. Bring to a simmer.

4. Cook for 15 minutes to allow flavors to meld.

5. Adjust seasoning if needed and garnish with fresh parsley before serving.

Nutritional Information (per cup):

- Calories: 220
- Protein: 10g
- Carbohydrates: 35g
- Dietary Fiber: 6g
- Fat: 5g
- Saturated Fat: 0.5g
- Sodium: 480mg
- Potassium: 560mg
- Phosphorus: 150mg

Cauliflower and Turmeric Soup

A vibrant and anti-inflammatory soup featuring cauliflower and turmeric, providing a delicious and health-conscious option.

Prep Time: 15 minutes

Cooking Time: 25 minutes

Serving Size: 1 cup

Ingredients:

- 1 small head cauliflower, chopped
- 1 onion, diced
- 2 cloves garlic, minced
- 1 teaspoon ground turmeric
- 6 cups low-sodium vegetable broth

- 1/2 cup coconut milk (light)
- Salt and pepper to taste
- 1 tablespoon coconut oil (optional)
- Fresh cilantro for garnish (optional)

Instructions:

1. In a pot, sauté diced onion and minced garlic in coconut oil until softened.

2. Add chopped cauliflower, ground turmeric, vegetable broth, coconut milk, salt, and pepper. Bring to a boil.

3. Reduce heat and simmer for 20 minutes or until cauliflower is tender.

4. Blend the soup until smooth using an immersion blender or regular blender.

5. Adjust seasoning if needed and garnish with fresh cilantro before serving.

Nutritional Information (per cup):

- Calories: 190
- Protein: 5g
- Carbohydrates: 30g
- Dietary Fiber: 8g
- Fat: 7g
- Saturated Fat: 5g
- Sodium: 520mg
- Potassium: 680mg

- Phosphorus: 160mg

Sweet Potato and Quinoa Chili

A hearty and nutritious chili featuring sweet potatoes, quinoa, and a medley of spices for a comforting and filling meal.

Prep Time: 20 minutes

Cooking Time: 30 minutes

Serving Size: 1.5 cup

Ingredients:

- 1 cup sweet potatoes, diced
- 1/2 cup quinoa, rinsed
- 1 can (15 oz) black beans, drained and rinsed
- 1 can (14 oz) diced tomatoes
- 1 onion, finely chopped
- 2 cloves garlic, minced
- 2 teaspoons chili powder
- 1 teaspoon cumin
- Salt and pepper to taste
- 4 cups low-sodium vegetable broth
- 1 tablespoon olive oil (optional)
- Greek yogurt and green onions for garnish (optional)

Instructions:

1. In a pot, sauté chopped onion and minced garlic in olive oil until translucent.

2. Add diced sweet potatoes, rinsed quinoa, black beans, diced tomatoes, chili powder, cumin, salt, and pepper. Bring to a simmer.

3. Cook for 25-30 minutes or until sweet potatoes and quinoa are cooked.

4. Adjust seasoning if needed and serve hot.

5. Garnish with a dollop of Greek yogurt and chopped green onions if desired.

Nutritional Information (per 1.5 cup):

- Calories: 300
- Protein: 12g
- Carbohydrates: 50g
- Dietary Fiber: 14g
- Fat: 5g
- Saturated Fat: 0.5g
- Sodium: 560mg
- Potassium: 900mg

SEA FOODS

Grilled Lemon Garlic Salmon

A flavorful and heart-healthy option, this grilled lemon garlic salmon is rich in omega-3 fatty acids and bursting with citrusy goodness.

Prep Time: 10 minutes

Marinating Time: 30 minutes

Cooking Time: 15 minutes

Serving Size: 1 fillet

Ingredients:

- 1 salmon fillet (6 oz)
- 1 lemon, juiced and zested
- 2 cloves garlic, minced
- 1 tablespoon olive oil
- 1 teaspoon dried dill
- Salt and pepper to taste

Instructions:

1. In a bowl, mix lemon juice, lemon zest, minced garlic, olive oil, dried dill, salt, and pepper.

2. Place the salmon fillet in a shallow dish and pour the marinade over it. Let it marinate in the refrigerator for 30 minutes.

3. Preheat the grill to medium-high heat.

4. Grill the salmon for 6-7 minutes per side or until it flakes easily with a fork.

5. Serve hot with your favorite side dishes.

Nutritional Information (per fillet):

- Calories: 320
- Protein: 34g
- Carbohydrates: 3g
- Dietary Fiber: 1g
- Fat: 20g
- Saturated Fat: 3g
- Sodium: 70mg
- Potassium: 850mg
- Phosphorus: 350mg

Baked Cod with Mediterranean Salsa

A light and vibrant dish featuring baked cod topped with a refreshing Mediterranean salsa for a burst of flavors.

Prep Time: 15 minutes

Cooking Time: 20 minutes

Serving Size: 1 fillet

Ingredients:

- 1 cod fillet (6 oz)
- 1 cup cherry tomatoes, halved
- 1/2 cucumber, diced

- 1/4 cup Kalamata olives, sliced

- 2 tablespoons red onion, finely chopped

- 2 tablespoons feta cheese, crumbled

- 1 tablespoon olive oil

- 1 tablespoon balsamic vinegar

- Fresh basil for garnish

Instructions:

1. Preheat the oven to 400°F (200°C).

2. Place the cod fillet on a baking sheet lined with parchment paper.

3. In a bowl, mix cherry tomatoes, cucumber, olives, red onion, feta cheese, olive oil, and balsamic vinegar to create the salsa.

4. Spoon the salsa over the cod fillet.

5. Bake for 15-20 minutes or until the cod is cooked through.

6. Garnish with fresh basil before serving.

Nutritional Information (per fillet):

- Calories: 280

- Protein: 25g

- Carbohydrates: 10g

- Dietary Fiber: 3g

- Fat: 15g

- Saturated Fat: 3g

- Sodium: 400mg

- Potassium: 650mg

- Phosphorus: 300mg

Shrimp Stir-Fry with Broccoli and Snow Peas

A quick and nutritious shrimp stir-fry featuring colorful vegetables, providing a low-calorie and high-protein option.

- *Prep Time: 15 minutes*

- *Cooking Time: 10 minutes*

- *Serving Size: 1 cup*

Ingredients:

- 1 cup shrimp, peeled and deveined

- 1 cup broccoli florets

- 1/2 cup snow peas, trimmed

- 1 carrot, julienned

- 2 cloves garlic, minced

- 1 tablespoon soy sauce (low-sodium)

- 1 tablespoon sesame oil

- 1 teaspoon ginger, grated

- Brown rice for serving

Instructions:

1. In a wok or skillet, heat sesame oil over medium-high heat.

2. Add shrimp and stir-fry for 2-3 minutes until they turn pink.

3. Add minced garlic and grated ginger, stir-frying for an additional 1 minute.

4. Add broccoli, snow peas, and julienned carrot. Continue stir-frying for 3-4 minutes until vegetables are tender-crisp.

5. Pour soy sauce over the mixture and stir to combine.

6. Serve the stir-fry over brown rice.

Nutritional Information (per cup):

- Calories: 250

- Protein: 20g

- Carbohydrates: 15g

- Dietary Fiber: 4g

- Fat: 10g

- Saturated Fat: 2g

- Sodium: 500mg

- Potassium: 450mg

- Phosphorus: 200mg

Lemon Herb Baked Tilapia

A light and zesty baked tilapia dish featuring a blend of fresh herbs and citrus for a delightful and heart-healthy option.

- *Prep Time: 10 minutes*

- *Cooking Time: 15 minutes*

- *Serving Size: 1 fillet*

Ingredients:

- 1 tilapia fillet (6 oz)

- 1 lemon, juiced and sliced

- 1 tablespoon fresh parsley, chopped

- 1 tablespoon fresh dill, chopped

- 1 tablespoon olive oil

- Salt and pepper to taste

Instructions:

1. Preheat the oven to 375°F (190°C).

2. Place the tilapia fillet on a baking sheet lined with parchment paper.

3. Drizzle olive oil over the fillet and season with salt and pepper.

4. Sprinkle chopped parsley and dill over the tilapia.

5. Squeeze lemon juice over the fillet and place lemon slices on top.

6. Bake for 12-15 minutes or until the tilapia is cooked through.

7. Serve with steamed vegetables or a side salad.

Nutritional Information (per fillet):

- Calories: 200
- Protein: 25g
- Carbohydrates: 2g
- Dietary Fiber: 1g
- Fat: 10g
- Saturated Fat: 1.5g
- Sodium: 80mg
- Potassium: 500mg
- Phosphorus: 220mg

Grilled Swordfish with Mango Salsa

A tropical-inspired dish featuring grilled swordfish topped with a refreshing mango salsa, offering a balance of flavors and nutrients.

- *Prep Time: 20 minutes*
- *Marinating Time: 30 minutes*
- *Cooking Time: 10 minutes*
- *Serving Size: 1 fillet*

Ingredients:

- 1 swordfish fillet (6 oz)
- 1 mango, diced
- 1/2 red bell pepper, diced
- 1/4 cup red onion, finely chopped
- 1 jalapeño, seeded and minced
- 2 tablespoons fresh cilantro, chopped
- 1 lime, juiced
- 1 tablespoon olive oil
- Salt and pepper to taste

Instructions:

1. In a bowl, mix diced mango, red bell pepper, red onion, jalapeño, cilantro, lime juice, olive oil, salt, and pepper to create the salsa.

2. Place the swordfish fillet in a shallow dish and pour half of the salsa over it. Let it marinate in the refrigerator for 30 minutes.

3. Preheat the grill to medium-high heat.

4. Grill the swordfish for 4-5 minutes per side or until it flakes easily with a fork.

5. Serve the grilled swordfish topped with the remaining mango salsa.

Nutritional Information (per fillet):

- Calories: 330
- Protein: 30g
- Carbohydrates: 20g
- Dietary Fiber: 3g
- Fat: 15g
- Saturated Fat: 2.5g
- Sodium: 90mg
- Potassium: 700mg
- Phosphorus: 300mg

Lemon Dijon Baked Scallops

A simple and elegant dish featuring baked scallops with a tangy lemon Dijon marinade for a burst of flavor without added calories.

- *Prep Time: 10 minutes*
- *Marinating Time: 15 minutes*
- *Cooking Time: 12 minutes*
- *Serving Size: 1/2 cup*

Ingredients:

- 1 cup scallops
- 1 lemon, juiced and zested
- 2 tablespoons Dijon mustard

- 1 tablespoon olive oil
- 1 clove garlic, minced
- 1 teaspoon fresh thyme, chopped
- Salt and pepper to taste

Instructions:

1. In a bowl, mix lemon juice, lemon zest, Dijon mustard, olive oil, minced garlic, fresh thyme, salt, and pepper to create the marinade.

2. Add scallops to the bowl and let them marinate for 15 minutes.

3. Preheat the oven to 400°F (200°C).

4. Place the scallops on a baking sheet lined with parchment paper.

5. Bake for 10-12 minutes or until scallops are opaque and cooked through.

6. Serve hot with a side of steamed vegetables or quinoa.

Nutritional Information (per 1/2 cup):

- Calories: 160
- Protein: 20g
- Carbohydrates: 5g
- Dietary Fiber: 1g
- Fat: 7g
- Saturated Fat: 1g
- Sodium: 350mg
- Potassium: 300mg

- Phosphorus: 180mg

Garlic Herb Grilled Shrimp Skewers

A quick and tasty option, these garlic herb grilled shrimp skewers are packed with protein and flavor, perfect for a light and satisfying meal.

- *Prep Time: 15 minutes*
- *Marinating Time: 30 minutes*
- *Cooking Time: 8 minutes*
- *Serving Size: 1 skewer*

Ingredients:

- 1 cup shrimp, peeled and deveined
- 2 cloves garlic, minced
- 1 tablespoon fresh parsley, chopped
- 1 tablespoon olive oil
- 1 teaspoon lemon zest
- 1/2 teaspoon dried oregano
- Salt and pepper to taste

Instructions:

1. In a bowl, mix minced garlic, chopped fresh parsley, olive oil, lemon zest, dried oregano, salt, and pepper to create the marinade.

2. Add shrimp to the bowl and let them marinate for 30 minutes.

3. Preheat the grill to medium-high heat.

4. Thread the marinated shrimp onto skewers.

5. Grill the shrimp skewers for 3-4 minutes per side or until they are opaque and cooked through.

6. Serve hot with a side of quinoa or a salad.

Nutritional Information (per skewer):

- Calories: 120

- Protein: 15g

- Carbohydrates: 1g

- Dietary Fiber: 0g

- Fat: 6g

- Saturated Fat: 1g

- Sodium: 180mg

- Potassium: 200mg

- Phosphorus: 140mg

Citrus Glazed Mahi-Mahi

A citrusy glaze enhances the flavor of this mahi-mahi dish, creating a light and satisfying meal that's quick and easy to prepare.

Prep Time: 10 minutes

Marinating Time: 15 minutes

Cooking Time: 12 minutes

Serving Size: 1 fillet

Ingredients:

- 1 mahi-mahi fillet (6 oz)

- 1 orange, juiced and zested

- 1 tablespoon honey

- 1 tablespoon soy sauce (low-sodium)

- 1 teaspoon fresh ginger, grated
- 1 tablespoon olive oil
- Sesame seeds for garnish (optional)

Instructions:

1. In a bowl, mix orange juice, orange zest, honey, soy sauce, grated ginger, and olive oil to create the marinade.

2. Place the mahi-mahi fillet in a shallow dish and pour the marinade over it. Let it marinate for 15 minutes.

3. Preheat the oven to 400°F (200°C).

4. Transfer the marinated mahi-mahi to a baking sheet lined with parchment paper.

5. Bake for 10-12 minutes or until the fish is cooked through.

6. Garnish with sesame seeds before serving.

Nutritional Information (per fillet):

- Calories: 290
- Protein: 30g
- Carbohydrates: 15g
- Dietary Fiber: 1g
- Fat: 12g
- Saturated Fat: 2g
- Sodium: 270mg
- Potassium: 650mg
- Phosphorus: 320mg

Cilantro Lime Grilled Halibut

A refreshing and herby dish featuring grilled halibut with a zesty cilantro lime marinade, providing a burst of freshness.

- *Prep Time: 15 minutes*
- *Marinating Time: 30 minutes*
- *Cooking Time: 12 minutes*
- *Serving Size: 1 fillet*

Ingredients:

- 1 halibut fillet (6 oz)
- 1 lime, juiced and zested
- 2 tablespoons fresh cilantro, chopped
- 1 tablespoon olive oil
- 1 teaspoon honey
- 1 clove garlic, minced
- Salt and pepper to taste

Instructions:

1. In a bowl, mix lime juice, lime zest, chopped cilantro, olive oil, honey, minced garlic, salt, and pepper to create the marinade.

2. Place the halibut fillet in a shallow dish and pour the marinade over it. Let it marinate for 30 minutes.

3. Preheat the grill to medium-high heat.

4. Grill the halibut for 6-7 minutes per side or until it flakes easily with a fork.

5. Serve hot with a side of steamed asparagus or quinoa.

Nutritional Information (per fillet):

- Calories: 280

- Protein: 28g

- Carbohydrates: 8g

- Dietary Fiber: 1g

- Fat: 15g

- Saturated Fat: 2.5g

- Sodium: 300mg

- Potassium: 600mg

- Phosphorus: 280mg

Teriyaki Glazed Tuna Steaks

A savory and slightly sweet teriyaki glaze enhances the flavor of these tuna steaks, providing a protein-packed and satisfying meal.

- *Prep Time: 10 minutes*

- *Marinating Time: 30 minutes*

- *Cooking Time: 8 minutes*

- *Serving Size: 1 steak*

Ingredients:

- 1 tuna steak (6 oz)

- 2 tablespoons low-sodium teriyaki sauce

- 1 tablespoon sesame oil

- 1 teaspoon fresh ginger, grated

- 1 tablespoon green onions, sliced

- Sesame seeds for garnish (optional)

Instructions:

1. In a bowl, mix teriyaki sauce, sesame oil, grated ginger, and sliced green onions to create the marinade.

2. Place the tuna steak in a shallow dish and pour the marinade over it. Let it marinate for 30 minutes.

3. Preheat the grill to medium-high heat.

4. Grill the tuna steak for 3-4 minutes per side for a medium-rare doneness.

5. Garnish with sesame seeds before serving.

Nutritional Information (per steak):

- Calories: 250
- Protein: 30g
- Carbohydrates: 5g
- Dietary Fiber: 0g
- Fat: 12g
- Saturated Fat: 2g
- Sodium: 350mg
- Potassium: 500mg
- Phosphorus: 300mg

MEAT AND POULTRY FOOD

Herb-Roasted Chicken Breast

A heart-healthy twist on classic roasted chicken. Herb-infused and oven-baked, this dish is both flavorful and nutritious.

- *Prep Time: 15 minutes*
- *Cooking Time: 30 minutes*
- *Serving Size: 1 chicken breast*

Ingredients:

- 1 boneless, skinless chicken breast (6 oz)
- 1 tablespoon olive oil
- 1 teaspoon dried rosemary
- 1 teaspoon dried thyme
- 1 teaspoon garlic powder
- Salt and pepper to taste

Instructions:

1. Preheat the oven to 400°F (200°C).
2. Rub the chicken breast with olive oil, dried rosemary, dried thyme, garlic powder, salt, and pepper.
3. Place the seasoned chicken breast on a baking sheet lined with parchment paper.
4. Bake for 25-30 minutes or until the internal temperature reaches 165°F (74°C).
5. Let it rest for a few minutes before slicing.
6. Serve with steamed vegetables or a side salad.

Nutritional Information (per chicken breast):

- Calories: 300
- Protein: 40g
- Carbohydrates: 0g
- Dietary Fiber: 0g
- Fat: 15g
- Saturated Fat: 3g
- Sodium: 90mg
- Potassium: 450mg
- Phosphorus: 300mg

Turkey and Vegetable Stir-Fry

A quick and nutritious stir-fry featuring lean ground turkey and an assortment of colorful vegetables, providing a balanced and satisfying meal.

- *Prep Time: 20 minutes*
- *Cooking Time: 15 minutes*
- *Serving Size: 1 cup*

Ingredients:

- 1 cup lean ground turkey
- 1 cup broccoli florets
- 1/2 cup bell peppers, sliced
- 1/2 cup carrots, julienned
- 2 cloves garlic, minced
- 1 tablespoon low-sodium soy sauce
- 1 tablespoon sesame oil

- 1 teaspoon ginger, grated
- Brown rice for serving

Instructions:

1. In a skillet, brown the ground turkey over medium-high heat.
2. Add minced garlic and grated ginger, stirring for 1-2 minutes.
3. Add broccoli, bell peppers, and julienned carrots. Continue stir-frying until vegetables are tender-crisp.
4. Pour soy sauce and sesame oil over the mixture, stirring to combine.
5. Serve the stir-fry over brown rice.

Nutritional Information (per cup):

- Calories: 250
- Protein: 30g
- Carbohydrates: 15g
- Dietary Fiber: 4g
- Fat: 10g
- Saturated Fat: 2g
- Sodium: 450mg
- Potassium: 500mg
- Phosphorus: 220mg

Lemon Garlic Grilled Turkey Cutlets

A zesty and light option featuring grilled turkey cutlets marinated in a flavorful blend of lemon and garlic.

- *Prep Time: 15 minutes*
- *Marinating Time: 30 minutes*

- *Cooking Time: 10 minutes*
- *Serving Size: 1 cutlet*

Ingredients:

- 1 turkey cutlet (6 oz)
- 1 lemon, juiced and zested
- 2 cloves garlic, minced
- 1 tablespoon olive oil
- 1 teaspoon dried oregano
- Salt and pepper to taste

Instructions:

1. In a bowl, mix lemon juice, lemon zest, minced garlic, olive oil, dried oregano, salt, and pepper.
2. Place the turkey cutlet in a shallow dish and pour the marinade over it. Let it marinate in the refrigerator for 30 minutes.
3. Preheat the grill to medium-high heat.
4. Grill the turkey cutlet for 4-5 minutes per side or until it reaches an internal temperature of 165°F (74°C).
5. Let it rest before slicing.
6. Serve with a side of quinoa or roasted vegetables.

Nutritional Information (per cutlet):

- Calories: 280
- Protein: 30g
- Carbohydrates: 2g
- Dietary Fiber: 0g
- Fat: 15g
- Saturated Fat: 2.5g

- Sodium: 100mg

- Potassium: 350mg

- Phosphorus: 280mg

Herb-Crusted Baked Pork Tenderloin

A succulent and herb-infused pork tenderloin, oven-baked to perfection for a flavorful and lean protein option.

- *Prep Time: 15 minutes*

- *Cooking Time: 25 minutes*

- *Serving Size: 3 oz*

Ingredients:

- 1 pork tenderloin (12 oz)

- 1 tablespoon Dijon mustard

- 1 tablespoon fresh rosemary, chopped

- 1 tablespoon fresh thyme, chopped

- 1 tablespoon whole-grain mustard

- Salt and pepper to taste

Instructions:

1. Preheat the oven to 400°F (200°C).

2. In a small bowl, mix Dijon mustard, fresh rosemary, fresh thyme, whole-grain mustard, salt, and pepper.

3. Rub the pork tenderloin with the herb-mustard mixture.

4. Place the pork tenderloin on a baking sheet lined with parchment paper.

5. Bake for 20-25 minutes or until the internal temperature reaches 145°F (63°C).

6. Let it rest for 5 minutes before slicing.

7. Serve with a side of roasted sweet potatoes or green beans.

Nutritional Information (per 3 oz):

- Calories: 150

- Protein: 20g

- Carbohydrates: 1g

- Dietary Fiber: 0g

- Fat: 7g

- Saturated Fat: 2g

- Sodium: 180mg

- Potassium: 300mg

- Phosphorus: 200mg

Chicken and Quinoa Stuffed Bell Peppers

A wholesome and protein-packed dish featuring a filling of lean ground chicken, quinoa, and vegetables, baked in colorful bell peppers.

- *Prep Time: 30 minutes*

- *Cooking Time: 35 minutes*

- *Serving Size: 1 stuffed pepper*

Ingredients:

- 1 bell pepper, halved and cleaned

- 1/2 cup lean ground chicken

- 1/4 cup cooked quinoa

- 1/4 cup black beans, drained and rinsed

- 1/4 cup corn kernels

- 1/4 cup diced tomatoes

- 1/4 teaspoon cumin

- 1/4 teaspoon chili powder

- Salt and pepper to taste

- 1 tablespoon fresh cilantro, chopped

Instructions:

1. Preheat the oven to 375°F (190°C).

2. In a skillet, cook lean ground chicken until browned.

3. In a bowl, combine cooked chicken, quinoa, black beans, corn, diced tomatoes, cumin, chili powder, salt, and pepper.

4. Stuff each bell pepper half with the chicken and quinoa mixture.

5. Place the stuffed peppers in a baking dish and bake for 30-35 minutes or until peppers are tender.

6. Garnish with fresh cilantro before serving.

Nutritional Information (per stuffed pepper):

- Calories: 200

- Protein: 18g

- Carbohydrates: 20g

- Dietary Fiber: 4g

- Fat: 6g

- Saturated Fat: 1.5g

- Sodium: 250mg

- Potassium: 450mg

- Phosphorus: 220Mg

Rosemary Garlic Grilled Lamb Chops

A sophisticated yet simple dish featuring grilled lamb chops marinated in rosemary and garlic for a burst of Mediterranean flavors.

- *Prep Time: 15 minutes*
- *Marinating Time: 30 minutes*
- *Cooking Time: 10 minutes*
- *Serving Size: 2 chops*

Ingredients:

- 4 lamb chops (8 oz)
- 2 tablespoons fresh rosemary, chopped
- 4 cloves garlic, minced
- 1 tablespoon olive oil
- Salt and pepper to taste

Instructions:

1. In a bowl, mix fresh rosemary, minced garlic, olive oil, salt, and pepper.
2. Rub the lamb chops with the rosemary-garlic mixture and let them marinate in the refrigerator for 30 minutes.
3. Preheat the grill to medium-high heat.
4. Grill the lamb chops for 4-5 minutes per side or until they reach the desired doneness.
5. Let them rest for a few minutes before serving.
6. Serve with a side of roasted vegetables or a quinoa salad.

Nutritional Information (per 2 chops):

- Calories: 400

- Protein: 40g

- Carbohydrates: 0g

- Dietary Fiber: 0g

- Fat: 25g

- Saturated Fat: 10g

- Sodium: 120mg

- Potassium: 550mg

- Phosphorus: 300mg

Lean Beef and Vegetable Skewers

A colorful and protein-packed dish featuring skewers with lean beef and a variety of vibrant vegetables, perfect for grilling or oven roasting.

- *Prep Time:20 minutes*

- *Cooking Time:15 minutes*

- *Serving Size:2 skewers*

Ingredients:

- 8 oz lean beef, cut into cubes

- 1 bell pepper, diced

- 1 zucchini, sliced

- 1 red onion, diced

- 1 tablespoon olive oil

- 1 teaspoon smoked paprika

- 1 teaspoon cumin

- Salt and pepper to taste

Instructions:

1. In a bowl, mix lean beef, diced bell pepper, sliced zucchini, diced red onion, olive oil, smoked paprika, cumin, salt, and pepper.

2. Thread the beef and vegetable pieces onto skewers.

3. Preheat the grill to medium-high heat.

4. Grill the skewers for 6-8 minutes, turning occasionally, until the beef is cooked to your liking.

5. Serve the skewers with a side of quinoa or a green salad.

Nutritional Information (per 2 skewers):

- Calories: 300
- Protein: 30g
- Carbohydrates: 10g
- Dietary Fiber: 3g
- Fat: 15g
- Saturated Fat: 4g
- Sodium: 200mg
- Potassium: 550mg
- Phosphorus: 280mg

Teriyaki Turkey Meatballs

A savory and lean option featuring turkey meatballs glazed in a delicious teriyaki sauce, perfect for a flavorful and satisfying meal.

- Prep Time:15 minutes
- Cooking Time:20 minutes
- Serving Size:5 meatballs

Ingredients:

- 1/2 lb lean ground turkey

- 1/4 cup whole wheat breadcrumbs

- 1/4 cup green onions, finely chopped

- 1 egg

- 2 tablespoons low-sodium teriyaki sauce

- 1 tablespoon sesame oil

- 1 teaspoon fresh ginger, grated

- 1 teaspoon garlic powder

Instructions:

1. Preheat the oven to 375°F (190°C).

2. In a bowl, mix lean ground turkey, whole wheat breadcrumbs, chopped green onions, egg, teriyaki sauce, sesame oil, grated ginger, and garlic powder.

3. Shape the mixture into meatballs and place them on a baking sheet lined with parchment paper.

4. Bake for 18-20 minutes or until the meatballs are cooked through.

5. Serve the meatballs with brown rice or steamed vegetables.

Nutritional Information (per 5 meatballs):

- Calories: 250

- Protein: 25g

- Carbohydrates: 15g

- Dietary Fiber: 2g

- Fat: 10g

- Saturated Fat: 2g

- Sodium: 400mg

- Potassium: 350mg

- Phosphorus: 220mg

Chicken and Lentil Curry

A hearty and flavorful curry featuring lean chicken and protein-rich lentils, simmered in a fragrant blend of spices.

- *Prep Time:20 minutes*

- *Cooking Time:30 minutes*

- *Serving Size: 1 cup*

Ingredients:

- 1 cup lean chicken breast, diced

- 1/2 cup dried lentils, rinsed and drained

- 1 cup tomatoes, diced

- 1 onion, finely chopped

- 2 cloves garlic, minced

- 1 tablespoon curry powder

- 1 teaspoon turmeric

- 1 teaspoon cumin

- 1/2 teaspoon chili powder

- 1/2 cup low-fat coconut milk

- Fresh cilantro for garnish

Instructions:

1. In a pot, sauté diced chicken, chopped onion, and minced garlic until chicken is browned.

2. Add diced tomatoes, dried lentils, curry powder, turmeric, cumin, chili powder, and low-fat coconut milk. Stir to combine.

3. Simmer the curry over medium heat for 25-30 minutes or until lentils are tender and chicken is cooked through.

4. Garnish with fresh cilantro before serving.

5. Serve the curry with brown rice or quinoa.

Nutritional Information (per cup):

- Calories: 300

- Protein: 25g

- Carbohydrates: 30g

- Dietary Fiber: 8g

- Fat: 8g

- Saturated Fat: 2g

- Sodium: 400mg

- Potassium: 600mg

- Phosphorus: 320mg

Grilled Chicken Caesar Salad

A classic Caesar salad with a heart-healthy twist, featuring grilled chicken breast and a lightened-up Caesar dressing.

- *Prep Time:15 minutes*

- *Cooking Time:15 minutes*

- *Serving Size:2 cups*

Ingredients:

- 2 boneless, skinless chicken breasts (8 oz each)

- 1 tablespoon olive oil

- Salt and pepper to taste

- 1 head romaine lettuce, chopped

- 1/4 cup grated Parmesan cheese
- Whole wheat croutons
- Caesar dressing (light)

Instructions:

1. Preheat the grill to medium-high heat.
2. Rub the chicken breasts with olive oil, salt, and pepper.
3. Grill the chicken for 6-8 minutes per side or until the internal temperature reaches 165°F (74°C).
4. Let the chicken rest before slicing.
5. In a large bowl, combine chopped romaine lettuce, grated Parmesan cheese, whole wheat croutons, and grilled chicken slices.
6. Drizzle with light Caesar dressing and toss to coat.
7. Serve the grilled chicken Caesar salad as a satisfying and heart-healthy meal.

Nutritional Information (per 2 cup):

- Calories: 350
- Protein: 30g
- Carbohydrates: 15g
- Dietary Fiber: 6g
- Fat: 18g
- Saturated Fat: 4g
- Sodium: 450mg
- Potassium: 700mg
- Phosphorus: 320mg

SMOOTHIE

Berry Bliss Smoothie

A refreshing blend of antioxidant-rich berries, perfect for a heart-healthy start to your day.

- Prep Time: 5 minutes
- Serving Size: 1 cup

Ingredients:

- 1/2 cup blueberries (fresh or frozen)
- 1/2 cup strawberries (fresh or frozen)
- 1/4 cup raspberries (fresh or frozen)
- 1/2 banana
- 1/2 cup low-fat yogurt
- 1/2 cup almond milk (unsweetened)

Instructions:

1. Combine blueberries, strawberries, raspberries, banana, low-fat yogurt, and almond milk in a blender.
2. Blend until smooth and creamy.
3. Pour into a glass and enjoy the burst of berry goodness.

Nutritional Information (per cup):

- Calories: 150
- Protein: 5g
- Carbohydrates: 30g
- Dietary Fiber: 7g
- Fat: 2g

- Saturated Fat: 0.5g

- Sodium: 40mg

- Potassium: 320mg

- Phosphorus: 120mg

Green Goddess Detox Smoothie

Packed with leafy greens and hydrating cucumber, this smoothie is a nutrient powerhouse for your heart.

- Prep Time: 7 minutes

- Serving Size: 1 cup

Ingredients:

- 1 cup spinach (fresh)

- 1/2 cucumber, peeled and sliced

- 1/2 green apple, cored and chopped

- 1/2 lemon, juiced

- 1/2 cup parsley (fresh)

- 1/2 cup coconut water (unsweetened)

Instructions:

1. Combine spinach, cucumber, green apple, lemon juice, parsley, and coconut water in a blender.

2. Blend until the mixture reaches a smooth consistency.

3. Pour into a glass, and relish the vibrant, heart-healthy goodness.

Nutritional Information (per cup):

- Calories: 120

- Protein: 4g

- Carbohydrates: 25g

- Dietary Fiber: 6g

- Fat: 1g

- Saturated Fat: 0g

- Sodium: 30mg

- Potassium: 420mg

- Phosphorus: 100mg

Tropical Paradise Smoothie

A delightful tropical blend that transports you to paradise while nourishing your heart.

- Prep Time: 8 minutes

- Serving Size: 1 cup

Ingredients:

- 1/2 cup pineapple chunks

- 1/2 cup mango chunks

- 1/2 banana

- 1/2 cup Greek yogurt (unsweetened)

- 1/2 cup coconut water (unsweetened)

- Ice cubes (optional)

Instructions:

1. Combine pineapple chunks, mango chunks, banana, Greek yogurt, and coconut water in a blender.

2. Add ice cubes if desired and blend until smooth.

3. Pour into a glass and savor the tropical flavors.

Nutritional Information (per cup):

- Calories: 160

- Protein: 7g

- Carbohydrates: 30g

- Dietary Fiber: 4g

- Fat: 2g

- Saturated Fat: 1g

- Sodium: 40mg

- Potassium: 350mg

- Phosphorus: 130mg

Heart-Healing Citrus Smoothie

A zesty and invigorating blend of citrus fruits, promoting heart health with a burst of vitamin C.

- Prep Time: 6 minutes

- Serving Size: 1 cup

Ingredients:

- 1/2 orange, peeled and segmented

- 1/2 grapefruit, peeled and segmented

- 1/2 lemon, juiced

- 1/2 cup low-fat yogurt

- 1/2 cup almond milk (unsweetened)

Instructions:

1. Combine orange segments, grapefruit segments, lemon juice, low-fat yogurt, and almond milk in a blender.

2. Blend until smooth and citrusy.

3. Pour into a glass and enjoy the zingy flavors.

Nutritional Information (per cup):

- Calories: 140

- Protein: 6g

- Carbohydrates: 28g

- Dietary Fiber: 5g

- Fat: 2g

- Saturated Fat: 0.5g

- Sodium: 45mg

- Potassium: 300mg

- Phosphorus: 110mg

Oatmeal Cookie Smoothie

A heart-healthy twist on a classic treat, blending the goodness of oats, cinnamon, and banana.

- Prep Time: 8 minutes

- Serving Size: 1 cup

Ingredients:

- 1/2 cup old-fashioned oats

- 1/2 banana

- 1/2 teaspoon ground cinnamon

- 1/2 cup low-fat milk

- 1/2 cup Greek yogurt (unsweetened)

- 1 tablespoon almond butter

Instructions:

1. Combine old-fashioned oats, banana, ground cinnamon, low-fat milk, Greek yogurt, and almond butter in a blender.

2. Blend until the mixture reaches a smooth consistency.

3. Pour into a glass and relish the wholesome taste of an oatmeal cookie.

Nutritional Information (per cup):

- Calories: 180
- Protein: 9g
- Carbohydrates: 30g
- Dietary Fiber: 5g
- Fat: 4g
- Saturated Fat: 1g
- Sodium: 55mg
- Potassium: 320mg
- Phosphorus: 180mg

Avocado Green Smoothie

A creamy and heart-healthy concoction featuring the goodness of avocado and leafy greens.

- Prep Time: 7 minutes
- Serving Size: 1 cup

Ingredients:

- 1/2 avocado
- 1/2 cup spinach (fresh)
- 1/2 cup kale (fresh)
- 1/2 banana
- 1/2 cup low-fat yogurt
- 1/2 cup coconut water (unsweetened)

Instructions:

1. Combine avocado, spinach, kale, banana, low-fat yogurt, and coconut water in a blender.
2. Blend until smooth and velvety.

3. Pour into a glass and savor the rich, green goodness.

Nutritional Information (per cup):

- Calories: 200
- Protein: 7g
- Carbohydrates: 25g
- Dietary Fiber: 8g
- Fat: 10g
- Saturated Fat: 2g
- Sodium: 50mg
- Potassium: 500mg
- Phosphorus: 150mg

Pomegranate Paradise Smoothie

An antioxidant-rich blend of pomegranate and berries, promoting heart health with every sip.

- Prep Time: 6 minutes
- Serving Size: 1 cup

Ingredients:

- 1/2 cup pomegranate seeds
- 1/2 cup blueberries (fresh or frozen)
- 1/2 cup raspberries (fresh or frozen)
- 1/2 cup low-fat yogurt
- 1/2 cup almond milk (unsweetened)

Instructions:

1. Combine pomegranate seeds, blueberries, raspberries, low-fat yogurt, and almond milk in a blender.
2. Blend until the mixture achieves a vibrant, pink hue.

3. Pour into a glass and indulge in the fruity paradise.

Nutritional Information (per cup):

- Calories: 160
- Protein: 6g
- Carbohydrates: 30g
- Dietary Fiber: 7g
- Fat: 3g
- Saturated Fat: 1g
- Sodium: 40mg
- Potassium: 280mg
- Phosphorus: 120mg

Banana Walnut Delight Smoothie

A heart-healthy blend featuring the natural sweetness of bananas and the crunch of walnuts.

- Prep Time: 5 minutes
- Serving Size: 1 cup

Ingredients:

- 1/2 banana
- 1/4 cup walnuts
- 1/2 cup low-fat yogurt
- 1/2 cup almond milk (unsweetened)
- 1/2 teaspoon vanilla extract
- Ice cubes (optional)

Instructions:

1. Combine banana, walnuts, low-fat yogurt, almond milk, vanilla extract, and ice cubes (if desired) in a blender.

2. Blend until smooth, with a delightful nutty texture.

3. Pour into a glass and relish the banana walnut delight.

Nutritional Information (per cup):

- Calories: 180
- Protein: 6g
- Carbohydrates: 25g
- Dietary Fiber: 4g
- Fat: 8g
- Saturated Fat: 1g
- Sodium: 35mg
- Potassium: 320mg
- Phosphorus: 130mg

Cocoa Berry Blast Smoothie

A decadent yet heart-healthy combination of antioxidant-rich berries and the rich flavor of cocoa.

- Prep Time: 8 minutes
- Serving Size: 1 cup

Ingredients:

- 1/2 cup mixed berries (blueberries, strawberries, raspberries)
- 1/2 banana
- 1 tablespoon unsweetened cocoa powder
- 1/2 cup low-fat yogurt
- 1/2 cup almond milk (unsweetened)

Instructions:

1. Combine mixed berries, banana, unsweetened cocoa powder, low-fat yogurt, and almond milk in a blender.
2. Blend until the cocoa berry blast reaches a smooth consistency.
3. Pour into a glass and relish the chocolate-infused goodness.

Nutritional Information (per cup):

- Calories: 170
- Protein: 7g
- Carbohydrates: 30g
- Dietary Fiber: 6g
- Fat: 4g
- Saturated Fat: 1g
- Sodium: 45mg
- Potassium: 300mg
- Phosphorus: 120mg

Spinach Mango Tango Smoothie

An energizing blend of tropical sweetness and nutrient-packed spinach for a heart-healthy dance of flavors.

- Prep Time: 7 minutes
- Serving Size: 1 cup

Ingredients:

- 1/2 cup mango chunks
- 1/2 banana
- 1/2 cup spinach (fresh)

- 1/2 cup low-fat yogurt

- 1/2 cup coconut water (unsweetened)

Instructions:

1. Combine mango chunks, banana, fresh spinach, low-fat yogurt, and coconut water in a blender.

2. Blend until the spinach mango tango achieves a vibrant green color.

3. Pour into a glass and enjoy the tropical dance of flavors.

Nutritional Information (per cup):

- Calories: 150

- Protein: 6g

- Carbohydrates: 30g

- Dietary Fiber: 5g

- Fat: 2g

- Saturated Fat: 1g

- Sodium: 40mg

- Potassium: 350mg

- Phosphorus: 100mg

These heart-healthy smoothie recipes offer a delightful fusion of flavors while prioritizing your cardiovascular well-being. Incorporate them into your daily routine to embark on a tasty journey towards a healthier heart.

SALADS

Mediterranean Quinoa Salad

This vibrant and heart-healthy salad brings together the goodness of quinoa, fresh vegetables, and a zesty dressing.

- Prep Time: 15 minutes
- Cooking Time: 15 minutes
- Serving Size: 1.5 cups

Ingredients:

- 1 cup cooked quinoa
- 1/2 cup cherry tomatoes, halved
- 1/2 cucumber, diced
- 1/4 cup red bell pepper, chopped
- 1/4 cup feta cheese, crumbled
- 2 tablespoons Kalamata olives, sliced
- 1 tablespoon red onion, finely chopped

Instructions:

1. In a large bowl, combine cooked quinoa, cherry tomatoes, cucumber, red bell pepper, feta cheese, olives, and red onion.
2. Toss the ingredients together until well mixed.
3. Drizzle with your favorite Mediterranean dressing and toss again before serving.

Nutritional Information (per serving):

- Calories: 300
- Protein: 10g

- Carbohydrates: 40g

- Dietary Fiber: 6g

- Fat: 12g

- Saturated Fat: 4g

- Sodium: 350mg

- Potassium: 480mg

- Phosphorus: 220mg

Grilled Chicken and Avocado Salad

A protein-packed salad featuring grilled chicken, creamy avocado, and a medley of fresh vegetables.

- Prep Time: 20 minutes

- Cooking Time: 15 minutes\

- Serving Size: 2 cups

Ingredients:

- 1 boneless, skinless chicken breast

- 1 avocado, sliced

- 2 cups mixed greens

- 1 cup cherry tomatoes, halved

- 1/2 cup cucumber, sliced

- 1/4 cup red onion, thinly sliced

- 2 tablespoons balsamic vinaigrette dressing

Instructions:

1. Season the chicken breast with salt and pepper, then grill until fully cooked.

2. Slice the grilled chicken into strips.

3. In a large bowl, combine mixed greens, cherry tomatoes, cucumber, red onion, and grilled chicken.

4. Top with sliced avocado and drizzle with balsamic vinaigrette.

Nutritional Information (per serving):

- Calories: 320
- Protein: 25g
- Carbohydrates: 15g
- Dietary Fiber: 7g
- Fat: 18g
- Saturated Fat: 3g
- Sodium: 450mg
- Potassium: 760mg
- Phosphorus: 300mg

Quinoa and Black Bean Salad

A hearty and protein-rich salad combining quinoa, black beans, and fresh vegetables for a satisfying meal.

- Prep Time: 15 minutes
- Cooking Time: 15 minutes (for quinoa)
- Serving Size: 1.5 cups

Ingredients:

- 1/2 cup cooked quinoa
- 1/2 cup black beans, canned and drained
- 1/2 cup corn kernels
- 1/4 cup red bell pepper, diced
- 1/4 cup cilantro, chopped

- 1/4 cup green onions, sliced

- Juice of 1 lime

- 1 tablespoon olive oil

- Salt and pepper to taste

Instructions:

1. Cook quinoa according to package instructions and let it cool.

2. In a large bowl, combine cooked quinoa, black beans, corn, red bell pepper, cilantro, and green onions.

3. In a small bowl, whisk together lime juice, olive oil, salt, and pepper.

4. Pour the dressing over the salad and toss gently to combine.

Nutritional Information (per serving):

- Calories: 280

- Protein: 10g

- Carbohydrates: 45g

- Dietary Fiber: 8g

- Fat: 7g

- Saturated Fat: 1g

- Sodium: 320mg

- Potassium: 550mg

- Phosphorus: 180mg

Salmon and Quinoa Salad

An omega-3 rich salad featuring grilled salmon, quinoa, and a variety of colorful vegetables.

- Prep Time: 20 minutes

- Cooking Time: 15 minutes (for quinoa and salmon)
- Serving Size: 1.5 cup

Ingredients:

- 1/2 cup cooked quinoa
- 4 ounces salmon fillet, grilled and flaked
- 1/2 cup cherry tomatoes, halved
- 1/4 cup cucumber, diced
- 1/4 cup red onion, finely chopped
- 1/4 cup bell peppers, mixed colors, diced
- 1 tablespoon fresh dill, chopped
- Juice of 1 lemon
- 1 tablespoon olive oil
- Salt and pepper to taste

Instructions:

1. Cook quinoa according to package instructions and let it cool.
2. Season the salmon fillet with salt and pepper, then grill until fully cooked. Flake the salmon.
3. In a large bowl, combine cooked quinoa, flaked salmon, cherry tomatoes, cucumber, red onion, bell peppers, and dill.
4. In a small bowl, whisk together lemon juice, olive oil, salt, and pepper. Pour over the salad and toss gently.

Nutritional Information (per serving):

- Calories: 350
- Protein: 25g
- Carbohydrates: 30g
- Dietary Fiber: 5g

- Fat: 16g

- Saturated Fat: 2.5g

- Sodium: 450mg

- Potassium: 680mg

- Phosphorus: 300mg

Chickpea and Spinach Salad

A plant-based delight featuring chickpeas, spinach, and a zesty tahini dressing.

- Prep Time: 15 minutes

- Cooking Time: No cooking required

- Serving Size: 1.5 cups

Ingredients:

- 1 cup canned chickpeas, drained and rinsed

- 2 cups fresh spinach leaves

- 1/4 cup cherry tomatoes, halved

- 1/4 cup cucumber, sliced

- 1/4 cup red bell pepper, diced

- 2 tablespoons red onion, finely chopped

- 1 tablespoon tahini

- Juice of 1 lemon

- 1 clove garlic, minced

- Salt and pepper to taste

Instructions:

1. In a large bowl, combine chickpeas, spinach, cherry tomatoes, cucumber, red bell pepper, and red onion.

2. In a small bowl, whisk together tahini, lemon juice, minced garlic, salt, and pepper.

3. Pour the dressing over the salad and toss gently to coat.

Nutritional Information (per serving):

- Calories: 280
- Protein: 12g
- Carbohydrates: 40g
- Dietary Fiber: 10g
- Fat: 10g
- Saturated Fat: 1g
- Sodium: 380mg
- Potassium: 620mg
- Phosphorus: 220mg

Quinoa and Chickpea Buddha Bowl

A nourishing bowl featuring quinoa, chickpeas, and an assortment of colorful vegetables, topped with a creamy tahini dressing.

- Prep Time: 20 minutes
- Cooking Time: 15 minutes (for quinoa)
- Serving Size: 2 cups

Ingredients:

- 1/2 cup cooked quinoa
- 1 cup canned chickpeas, drained and rinsed
- 1 cup kale, chopped
- 1/2 cup carrot, grated
- 1/2 cup red cabbage, shredded

- 1/4 cup radishes, sliced

- 2 tablespoons pumpkin seeds

- 2 tablespoons tahini

- 1 tablespoon apple cider vinegar

- 1 tablespoon olive oil

- Salt and pepper to taste

Instructions:

1. Cook quinoa according to package instructions and let it cool.

2. In a large bowl, assemble quinoa, chickpeas, kale, carrot, red cabbage, and radishes.

3. In a small bowl, whisk together tahini, apple cider vinegar, olive oil, salt, and pepper.

4. Drizzle the dressing over the bowl and sprinkle with pumpkin seeds.

Nutritional Information (per serving):

- Calories: 320

- Protein: 14g

- Carbohydrates: 45g

- Dietary Fiber: 9g

- Fat: 12g

- Saturated Fat: 1.5g

- Sodium: 420mg

- Potassium: 750mg

- Phosphorus: 260mg

Shrimp and Avocado Salad

A refreshing salad featuring succulent shrimp, creamy avocado, and a citrusy dressing.

- Prep Time: 15 minutes
- Cooking Time: 5 minutes (for shrimp)
- Serving Size: 1.5 cups

Ingredients:

- 8 ounces shrimp, peeled and deveined
- 1 avocado, sliced
- 2 cups mixed salad greens
- 1/2 cup cherry tomatoes, halved
- 1/4 cup red onion, thinly sliced
- Juice of 1 lime
- 1 tablespoon olive oil
- 1 teaspoon Dijon mustard
- Salt and pepper to taste

Instructions:

1. In a pan, cook the shrimp with a sprinkle of salt and pepper until pink and opaque.
2. In a large bowl, combine mixed salad greens, cherry tomatoes, red onion, and sliced avocado.
3. Whisk together lime juice, olive oil, Dijon mustard, salt, and pepper for the dressing.
4. Add the cooked shrimp to the salad and drizzle with the citrusy dressing.

Nutritional Information (per serving):

- Calories: 280
- Protein: 20g
- Carbohydrates: 15g
- Dietary Fiber: 8g
- Fat: 16g
- Saturated Fat: 2.5g
- Sodium: 380mg
- Potassium: 660mg
- Phosphorus: 200mg

Spinach and Strawberry Salad

A delightful mix of fresh spinach, sweet strawberries, and crunchy almonds, topped with a balsamic vinaigrette.

- Prep Time: 10 minutes
- Cooking Time: No cooking required
- Serving Size: 1.5 cups

Ingredients:

- 2 cups fresh spinach leaves
- 1 cup strawberries, sliced
- 1/4 cup almonds, sliced
- 2 tablespoons feta cheese, crumbled
- 2 tablespoons balsamic vinaigrette dressing

Instructions:

1. In a large bowl, combine fresh spinach, sliced strawberries, almonds, and crumbled feta cheese.

2. Drizzle with balsamic vinaigrette and toss gently before serving.

Nutritional Information (per serving):

- Calories: 250
- Protein: 8g
- Carbohydrates: 20g
- Dietary Fiber: 6g
- Fat: 16g
- Saturated Fat: 2g
- Sodium: 320mg
- Potassium: 580mg
- Phosphorus: 170mg

Tuna and White Bean Salad

A protein-packed salad featuring tuna, white beans, and a zesty lemon dressing for a satisfying and nutritious meal.

- Prep Time: 15 minutes
- Cooking Time: No cooking required
- Serving Size: 1.5 cup

Ingredients:

- 1 can (5 ounces) tuna in water, drained
- 1 cup canned white beans, drained and rinsed
- 1/2 cup cherry tomatoes, halved
- 1/4 cup red onion, finely chopped
- 1/4 cup black olives, sliced
- 2 tablespoons parsley, chopped
- Juice of 1 lemon

- 1 tablespoon olive oil
- Salt and pepper to taste

Instructions:

1. In a large bowl, combine tuna, white beans, cherry tomatoes, red onion, black olives, and parsley.
2. In a small bowl, whisk together lemon juice, olive oil, salt, and pepper.
3. Pour the dressing over the salad and toss gently to combine.

Nutritional Information (per serving):

- Calories: 280
- Protein: 20g
- Carbohydrates: 20g
- Dietary Fiber: 6g
- Fat: 15g
- Saturated Fat: 2g
- Sodium: 480mg
- Potassium: 580mg
- Phosphorus: 250mg

Roasted Vegetable Quinoa Salad

A warm and hearty salad featuring roasted vegetables, quinoa, and a balsamic glaze for a burst of flavors.

- Prep Time: 20 minutes
- Cooking Time: 25 minutes (for roasting)
- Serving Size: 1.5 cup

Ingredients:

- 1 cup cooked quinoa
- 1 cup broccoli florets
- 1 cup cherry tomatoes
- 1/2 cup red bell pepper, sliced
- 1/4 cup red onion, thinly sliced
- 2 tablespoons balsamic glaze
- 1 tablespoon olive oil
- Salt and pepper to taste

Instructions:

1. Preheat the oven to 400°F (200°C).
2. In a baking sheet, toss broccoli, cherry tomatoes, red bell pepper, and red onion with olive oil, salt, and pepper.
3. Roast the vegetables for 25 minutes or until they are tender and slightly browned.
4. In a large bowl, combine cooked quinoa and the roasted vegetables.
5. Drizzle with balsamic glaze and toss gently before serving.

Nutritional Information (per serving):

- Calories: 320
- Protein: 10g
- Carbohydrates: 50g
- Dietary Fiber: 8g
- Fat: 10g
- Saturated Fat: 1.5g
- Sodium: 320mg

- Potassium: 690mg

- Phosphorus: 200mg

Enjoy these delicious and heart-healthy salad recipes, each crafted with a perfect balance of flavors and nutrients to support your overall well-being.

30 DAYS MEAL PLAN

Day 1:

- **Breakfast:** Berry-Almond Chia Pudding Parfait
- **Lunch:** Grilled Chicken Caesar Salad
- **Dinner:** Grilled Lemon Garlic Salmon
- **Smoothie:** Berry Bliss Smoothie
- *Tip: Boost your Omega-3 intake with salmon and add a handful of fresh berries to your salad for an antioxidant punch.*

Day 2:

- **Breakfast:** Greek Yogurt Parfait with Fruit and Granola
- **Lunch:** Quinoa and Black Bean Salad
- **Dinner:** Baked Cod with Mediterranean Salsa
- **Smoothie:** Green Goddess Detox Smoothie
- *Tip: Greek yogurt provides probiotics for gut health, and quinoa adds plant-based protein to your salad.*

Day 3:

- **Breakfast:** Vegetable and Egg Breakfast Burrito
- **Lunch:** Salmon and Quinoa Salad
- **Dinner:** Shrimp Stir-Fry with Broccoli and Snow Peas
- **Smoothie:** Tropical Paradise Smoothie
- *Tip: Choose colorful vegetables for your stir-fry to maximize vitamins and minerals.*

Day 4:

- **Breakfast:** Spinach and Mushroom Egg White Omelette
- **Lunch:** Quinoa and Chickpea Buddha Bowl

- **Dinner:** Lemon Herb Baked Tilapia
- **Smoothie:** Heart-Healing Citrus smoothie
- *Tip: Egg whites are a low-cholesterol source of protein, and quinoa adds a satisfying crunch to your bowl.*

Day 5:

- **Breakfast:** Quinoa and Berry Breakfast Bowl
- **Lunch:** Chickpea and Spinach Salad
- **Dinner:** Grilled Swordfish with Mango Salsa
- **Smoothie:** Oatmeal Cookie Smoothie
- *Tip: Berries in your breakfast bowl provide a sweet kick and antioxidants.*

Day 6:

- **Breakfast:** Avocado and Tomato Toast
- **Lunch:** Roasted Vegetable Quinoa Salad
- **Dinner:** Citrus Glazed Mahi-Mahi
- **Smoothie:** Avocado Green Smoothie
- *Tip: Avocado adds creamy texture and heart-healthy fats to your morning toast.*

Day 7:

- **Breakfast:** Blueberry and Almond Overnight Oats
- **Lunch:** Cilantro Lime Grilled Halibut
- **Dinner:** Teriyaki Glazed Tuna Steaks
- **Smoothie:** Pomegranate Paradise Smoothie
- *Tip: Overnight oats are a time-saving, fiber-rich breakfast option.*

Day 8:

- **Breakfast:** Whole Grain Pancakes with Berries
- **Lunch:** Shrimp and Avocado Salad
- **Dinner:** Garlic Herb Grilled Shrimp Skewers
- **Smoothie:** Banana Walnut Delight Smoothie
- *Tip: Whole grain pancakes provide sustained energy and are a delightful breakfast option.*

Day 9:

- **Breakfast:** Smoked Salmon and Avocado Bagel
- **Lunch:** Spinach and Strawberry Salad
- **Dinner:** Herb-Crusted Baked Pork Tenderloin
- **Smoothie:** Cocoa Berry Blast Smoothie
- *Tip: Add a handful of spinach to your salad for an iron and fiber boost.*

Day 10:

- **Breakfast:** Banana Walnut Breakfast Muffins
- **Lunch:** Tuna and White Bean Salad
- **Dinner:** Chicken and Quinoa Stuffed Bell Peppers
- **Smoothie:** Spinach Mango Tango Smoothie
- *Tip: Use ripe bananas for natural sweetness in your muffins.*

Day 11:

- **Breakfast:** Hearty Lentil and Vegetable Soup
- **Lunch:** Quinoa and Vegetable Stew
- **Dinner:** Rosemary Garlic Grilled Lamb Chops
- **Smoothie:** Berry Bliss Smoothie

- *Tip: Lentils are an excellent source of plant-based protein and fiber.*

Day 12:

- **Breakfast:** Tomato Basil Quinoa Soup
- **Lunch:** Lemon Garlic Grilled Turkey Cutlets
- **Dinner:** Lean Beef and Vegetable Skewers
- **Smoothie:** Green Goddess Detox Smoothie
- *Tip: Lean meats paired with colorful veggies make for a satisfying and heart-healthy meal.*

Day 13:

- **Breakfast:** Spinach and White Bean Soup
- **Lunch:** Herb-Roasted Chicken Breast
- **Dinner:** Teriyaki Turkey Meatballs
- **Smoothie:** Tropical Paradise Smoothie
- *Tip: White beans add a creamy texture to your soup and boost fiber content.*

Day 14:

- **Breakfast:** Butternut Squash and Red Lentil Soup
- **Lunch:** Chicken and Lentil Curry
- **Dinner:** Grilled Chicken and Avocado Salad
- **Smoothie:** Heart-Healing Citrus smoothie
- *Tip: Lentils and curry offer a flavorful, plant-based protein option.*

Day 15:

- **Breakfast:** Minestrone Soup with Whole Wheat Pasta
- **Lunch:** Quinoa and Chickpea Buddha Bowl

- **Dinner:** Grilled Swordfish with Mango Salsa
- **Smoothie:** Oatmeal Cookie Smoothie
- *Tip: Whole wheat pasta in your minestrone soup adds fiber for heart health.*

Day 16:

- **Breakfast:** Roasted Red Pepper and Chickpea Soup
- **Lunch:** Shrimp and Avocado Salad
- **Dinner:** Lemon Herb Baked Tilapia
- **Smoothie:** Avocado Green Smoothie
- *Tip: Chickpeas are a versatile and heart-healthy addition to your soup.*

Day 17:

- **Breakfast:** Quinoa and Vegetable Stew
- **Lunch:** Quinoa and Black Bean Salad
- **Dinner:** Citrus Glazed Mahi-Mahi
- **Smoothie:** Pomegranate Paradise Smoothie
- *Tip: Quinoa is a complete protein, providing all essential amino acids.*

Day 18:

- **Breakfast:** Lemon Garlic Orzo Soup
- **Lunch:** Salmon and Quinoa Salad
- **Dinner:** Teriyaki Glazed Tuna Steaks
- **Smoothie:** Banana Walnut Delight Smoothie
- *Tip: Orzo adds a delightful texture to your morning soup.*

Day 19:

- **Breakfast:** Cauliflower and Turmeric Soup

- **Lunch:** Chickpea and Spinach Salad
- **Dinner:** Garlic Herb Grilled Shrimp Skewers
- **Smoothie:** Cocoa Berry Blast Smoothie
- *Tip: Turmeric in your soup offers anti-inflammatory benefits.*

Day 20:

- **Breakfast:** Sweet Potato and Quinoa Chili
- **Lunch:** Roasted Vegetable Quinoa Salad
- **Dinner:** Cilantro Lime Grilled Halibut
- **Smoothie:** Spinach Mango Tango Smoothie
- *Tip: Sweet potatoes are rich in vitamins and add natural sweetness to your chili.*

Day 21:

- **Breakfast:** Grilled Lemon Garlic Salmon
- **Lunch:** Quinoa and Chickpea Buddha Bowl
- **Dinner:** Herb-Roasted Chicken Breast
- **Smoothie:** Berry Bliss Smoothie
- *Tip: Salmon provides Omega-3 fatty acids, promoting heart health.*

Day 22:

- **Breakfast:** Lemon Herb Baked Tilapia
- **Lunch:** Lean Beef and Vegetable Skewers
- **Dinner:** Rosemary Garlic Grilled Lamb Chops
- **Smoothie:** Green Goddess Detox Smoothie
- *Tip: Tilapia is a lean protein choice, and rosemary adds a fragrant touch to lamb.*

Day 23:

- **Breakfast:** Quinoa and Vegetable Stew
- **Lunch:** Teriyaki Turkey Meatballs
- **Dinner:** Grilled Chicken and Avocado Salad
- **Smoothie:** Tropical Paradise Smoothie
- *Tip: Turkey meatballs are a lean and flavorful option.*

Day 24:

- **Breakfast:** Butternut Squash and Red Lentil Soup
- **Lunch:** Grilled Swordfish with Mango Salsa
- **Dinner:** Chicken and Lentil Curry
- **Smoothie:** Heart-Healing Citrus smoothie
- *Tip: Lentils in your soup provide a plant-based protein source.*

Day 25:

- **Breakfast:** Minestrone Soup with Whole Wheat Pasta
- **Lunch:** Quinoa and Chickpea Buddha Bowl
- **Dinner:** Grilled Swordfish with Mango Salsa
- **Smoothie:** Oatmeal Cookie Smoothie
- *Tip: Whole wheat pasta adds a nutritional boost to your minestrone.*

Day 26:

- **Breakfast:** Roasted Red Pepper and Chickpea Soup
- **Lunch:** Lemon Herb Baked Tilapia
- **Dinner:** Teriyaki Glazed Tuna Steaks
- **Smoothie:** Avocado Green Smoothie
- *Tip: Chickpeas in your soup provide fiber and protein.*

Day 27:

- **Breakfast:** Quinoa and Vegetable Stew
- **Lunch:** Citrus Glazed Mahi-Mahi
- **Dinner:** Grilled Chicken and Avocado Salad
- **Smoothie:** Pomegranate Paradise Smoothie
- *Tip: Quinoa is a versatile grain that complements many dishes.*

Day 28:

- **Breakfast:** Lemon Garlic Orzo Soup
- **Lunch:** Teriyaki Turkey Meatballs
- **Dinner:** Garlic Herb Grilled Shrimp Skewers
- **Smoothie:** Banana Walnut Delight Smoothie
- *Tip: Orzo adds a delightful touch to your morning soup.*

Day 29:

- **Breakfast:** Cauliflower and Turmeric Soup
- **Lunch:** Garlic Herb Grilled Shrimp Skewers
- **Dinner:** Sweet Potato and Quinoa Chili
- **Smoothie:** Cocoa Berry Blast Smoothie
- *Tip: Turmeric in your soup has anti-inflammatory properties.*

Day 30:

- **Breakfast:** Sweet Potato and Quinoa Chili
- **Lunch:** Roasted Vegetable Quinoa Salad
- **Dinner:** Cilantro Lime Grilled Halibut
- **Smoothie:** Spinach Mango Tango Smoothie
- *Tip: Sweet potatoes add natural sweetness to your chili.*

Congratulations on completing the 30-day Heart Healthy Recipe Cookbook for Seniors meal plan! Remember to adjust portions based on individual needs and consult with a healthcare professional for personalized advice. Enjoy your heart-healthy journey!

CONCLUSION

In conclusion, embarking on the journey of understanding and prioritizing heart health for seniors has been an enlightening exploration. Throughout this comprehensive guide, we've delved into the nuances of a heart-healthy diet, unraveling the importance of key nutrients, mastering portion control, and deciphering the intricacies of food labels. We've ventured into the realm of building a heart-healthy pantry, exploring essential ingredients, cooking oils and fats, and honing smart grocery shopping tips. The culinary journey extended to the incorporation of wholesome elements like whole grains, lean proteins, vibrant vegetables, heart-boosting fruits, healthy fats, low-fat dairy, and an array of flavorful herbs and spices. We navigated the seas of fish and seafood, traversed the fields of legumes and high-fiber foods, and simmered in the nourishing world of low-sodium soups.

Understanding the basics of heart-healthy eating became more than just a dietary consideration; it evolved into a lifestyle centered around nourishing the body and soul. Key nutrients, portion control, and the ability to decipher food labels now serve as guiding principles in crafting meals that not only support cardiovascular health but also provide a delightful culinary experience.

The heart-healthy pantry emerged as the foundation of this nutritional journey. Armed with essential ingredients, an awareness of cooking oils and fats, and the wisdom of smart grocery shopping, individuals can stock their kitchens with the building blocks of nutritious, delicious meals. Whole grains, lean proteins, colorful vegetables, heart-healthy fruits, and an array of other elements form a palette of choices, inviting creativity and diversity into everyday eating.

Our exploration further extended to crafting delectable recipes, including nutrient-rich breakfast options, soul-soothing soups, heartwarming seafood dishes, and satisfying meat and poultry creations. Each recipe, meticulously detailed with preparation time, cooking time, serving size, ingredients, and comprehensive nutritional information, serves as a testament to the harmonious blend of flavor and nutrition.

Navigating the intricate landscape of sodium, we uncovered the importance of mindful consumption, particularly for seniors with heart conditions. The chapters dedicated to sodium and low-sodium options offered insights into maintaining a delicate balance, ensuring that flavor isn't compromised while safeguarding cardiovascular health.

As we immerse ourselves in this culinary and nutritional odyssey, it is crucial to reflect on the profound impact of our dietary choices. The 30-day meal plan, meticulously curated with a blend of breakfast delights, hearty lunches, and satisfying dinners, encapsulates the essence of a heart-healthy lifestyle. Each day's selection showcases the versatility of ingredients and the artistry of combining flavors to create meals that are not only good for the heart but also a joy to the palate.

In the pursuit of heart health, it's essential to recognize that this journey is not a sprint but a marathon. It involves commitment, adaptability, and a genuine desire for holistic well-being. The understanding gained from this guide empowers individuals to make informed choices, fostering a sense of control over their health destiny. It's not just about what's on the plate; it's about cultivating a mindful and nurturing relationship with food.

In the words of Hippocrates, the ancient Greek physician often hailed as the father of medicine, "Let food be thy medicine and medicine be thy food." This timeless wisdom encapsulates the essence of our exploration into heart-healthy living. By embracing the principles of nourishment, balance, and mindful consumption, we lay the foundation for a resilient heart and a vibrant life.

As you embark on your journey towards heart health, remember that every choice matters. The recipes, insights, and tips shared here are not mere guidelines but invitations to a lifestyle that cherishes the heart as the epicenter of well-being. May your culinary adventures continue to be infused with creativity, joy, and an unwavering commitment to a heart-healthy tomorrow.

www.ingramcontent.com/pod-product-compliance
Lightning Source LLC
Chambersburg PA
CBHW060015260726
48663CB00006B/191